Essentials of
Traumatic Injuries
to the Teeth

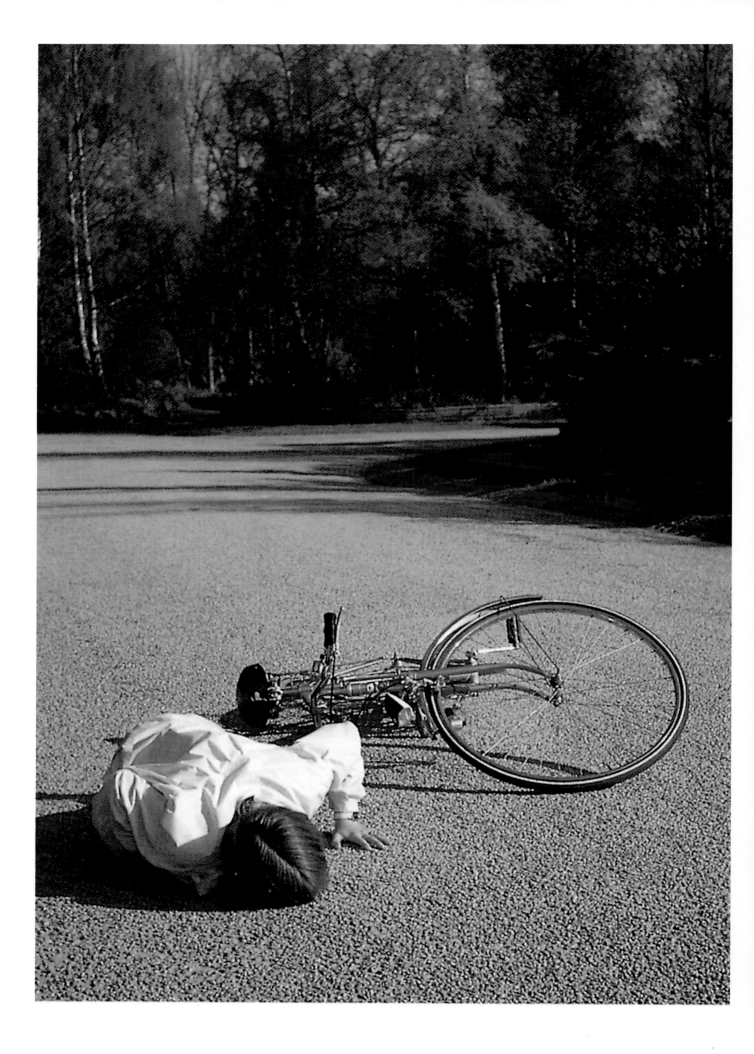

J.O. Andreasen and F.M. Andreasen

Essentials of Traumatic Injuries to the Teeth

A step-by-step treatment guide
Second Edition

Department of Oral and Maxillofacial Surgery
University Hospital (Rigshospitalet), Copenhagen, Denmark

Specialist consultant in Dental Trauma,
Copenhagen, Denmark

Blackwell
Munksgaard

© 2000 J.O. Andreasen, F.M. Andreasen and Munksgaard, Copenhagen

Blackwell Munksgaard, a Blackwell Publishing imprint
Editorial Offices:
Blackwell Publishing Ltd, 9600 Garsington Road, Oxford OX4 2DQ, UK
   Tel: +44 (0)1865 776868
Iowa State Press, a Blackwell Publishing Company, 2121 State Avenue,
   Ames, Iowa 50014-8300,USA Tel: 1 515 292 0140
Blackwell Publishing Asia, 550 Swanston Street, Carlton,Victoria 3053, Australia
   Tel. +61 (0)3 8359 1011

Second edition published 2000
Reprinted with minor revisions by Blackwell Munksgaard 2004

ISBN 87-16-12277-1

Medical illustrations by HDC design, Henning Dalhoff
Cover and lay-out by Henning Dalhoff
Typesetting by Special-Trykkeriet Viborg a-s
Reproduction by Gopsons Papers Limited

The publisher's policy is to use permanent paper from mills that operate a sustainable forestry policy, and which has been manufactured from pulp processed using acid-free and elementary chlorine-free practices. Futhermore, the publisher ensures that the text paper and cover board used have met acceptable environmental accreditation standards.

For further information on Blackwell Munksgaard, visit our website:
www.dentistry.blackwellmunksgaard.com

Contents

FOREWORD 7

CHAPTER 1 Examination of the traumatized patient,
wound healing and treatment principles . 9

CHAPTER 2 Crown fracture 21

CHAPTER 3 Crown-root fracture 47

CHAPTER 4 Root fracture 63

CHAPTER 5 Concussion and subluxation 77

CHAPTER 6 Extrusion and lateral luxation 85

CHAPTER 7 Intrusion 103

CHAPTER 8 Avulsion injury 113

CHAPTER 9 Fracture of the alveolar process 133

CHAPTER 10 Injuries to the primary dentition 141

CHAPTER 11 Soft tissue injuries 155

APPENDIX 1 Emergency record for acute dental
trauma 173

APPENDIX 2 Clinical examination form for the time of
injury and follow-up examinations 177

APPENDIX 3 Clinical and radiographic findings with
the various luxation types 178

APPENDIX 4 Summary of treatment and follow-up
procedures and recall schedule following
the various trauma types 179

BIBLIOGRAPHY 181

INDEX 186

Foreword

One feature common to all patients presenting with acute dental trauma is the fact that they come to us unexpectedly. There is no spot in our appointment books designated "*Trauma*." They just come. It can be in the midst of a busy day, where others are waiting patiently or impatiently for treatment; or in the middle of the night.

The purpose of this book is to provide the clinician, whether in a dental practice or emergency service of a hospital, with a readily accessible guide to initial treatment of acute dental trauma. In that regard, in order to facilitate initial examination and record-keeping, Appendix 1 provides a standardized emergency chart that can be used to guide the examiner through a complete trauma examination. Moreover, Appendix 2 provides a clinical examination form for acute and follow-up examinations. Appendix 3 summarizes the clinical and radiographic characteristics of each luxation category. It is suggested that these or similar forms be duplicated and completed as an integral part of the trauma patient's record.

In the case of some trauma entities, such as concussion, subluxation and some injuries to the primary dentition, observation "therapy" is the only treatment needed. In other situations, repositioning and splinting procedures characterize treatment. Techniques for the reduction of tooth dislocations include immediate repositioning or repositioning using an orthodontic or surgical approach. The decision of which procedure to employ will be discussed. Finally Appendix 4 is aimed at assisting in determining when the patient should be seen in order to detect changes in the follow-up period which might necessitate interceptive therapy.

It is the authors' hope that *Essential of Traumatic Injuries to the Teeth. A step-by-step treatment guide* will aid the dental clinician in providing optimal care to the acutely traumatized patient, thereby reducing the stress and anxiety of the first treatment episode – for both the patient and the clinician.

Those readers who are interested in an in-depth discussion of the biological impact of the various trauma entities upon the pulp and periodontium, the pathogenesis of the various healing complications and long-term effects and treatment of oral trauma, are referred to *Textbook and Color Atlas of Traumatic Injuries to the Teeth*.

Finally, the authors would like to express their gratitude to Drs. Miomir Cvek and Barbro Malmgren, Department of Pedodontics at the Eastman Dental Institute, Stockholm, Sweden, for their valuable contributions to the chapters on crown and crown-root fractures. We also thank the staff of the Department of Oral and Maxillofacial Surgery, University Hospital, Copenhagen.

In the second edition of *Essentials of Traumatic Dental Injuries* a revision of both text and illustrations has been made and new sections have been added dealing with healing subsequent to trauma, treatment procedures optimizing wound healing, and finally a description of diagnosis and treatment of the frequent associated soft tissue injuries involving gingiva, mucosa and/or skin.

Jens O. Andreasen   *Frances M. Andreasen*

Copenhagen, 2000

Examination of the traumatized patient, wound healing and treatment principles

EXAMINATION OF THE TRAUMATIZED PATIENT, WOUND HEALING AND TREATMENT PRINCIPLES

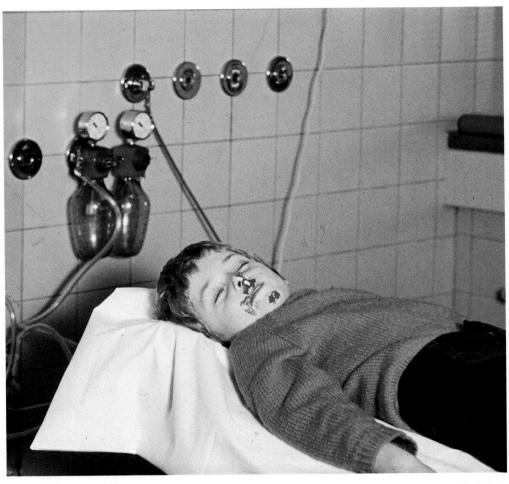

Fig. 1.1. **Examination of the injured patient**

CHAPTER 1

Examination of the traumatized patient

In order to arrive at a quick and correct diagnosis of the probable extent of injury to the pulp, periodontium and associated structures, a systematic examination of the traumatized patient is essential and will be demonstrated in the following.

When the patient is received for treatment of an acute trauma, the oral region is usually heavily contaminated (Fig. 1.1). The first step in the examination procedure, therefore, is to wash the patient's face. In case of soft tissue wounds, a mild detergent should be used (see later). While this is being done, it is possible to get an initial impression of the extent of injury. Thereafter, a series of questions must be asked to aid in diagnosis and treatment planning.

These questions include:

How did the injury occur? The answer will indicate the location of possible injury zones (e.g. crown-root fractures in the premolar and molar region after impacts under the chin) (Fig. 1.2).

Where did the injury occur? While there might be legal implications in the answer to this question, this will also indicate the possibility of contamination of wounds.

When did the injury occur? The answer will imply a time factor, which could influence the choice of treatment. This time factor becomes critical in the case of avulsed or displaced teeth.

Fig. 1.2. **Direction of impact**
The direction of impact determines the pattern of injury. A soft tissue bruise under the chin can imply a complicated injury pattern, often involving fractures of premolars and molars, the temporomandibular joint and symphysis, as well as risk of cerebral involvement.
In this case, a blow to the chin has resulted in multiple crown-root fractures of premolars.

Fig. 1.3. **Previous injury, primary dentition**
This 4-year-old girl has suffered subluxation of her right central incisor. At the age of 1 year there was an injury affecting both central incisors resulting in pulp necrosis of the right central incisor and pulp canal obliteration of the left incisor.

Finally any inconsistency between the appearance of the wounds on a child and the history supplied should raise the suspicion of the battered child syndrome. In this case, the patient should also be examined by a pediatrician.

Was there a period of unconsciousness? If so, for how long? Is there headache? amnesia? nausea? vomiting? These are all signs of brain concussion and require medical attention. However, this does not contraindicate emergency treatment of the dental injury. Early treatment will in most cases improve later prognosis.

Has there been previous injury to the teeth? Answers to this question may explain radiographic findings, such as pulp canal obliteration and incomplete root formation in a dentition with otherwise completed root development (Figs. 1.3 and 1.4).

Is there any disturbance in the bite? An affirmative answer can imply one of the following conditions: tooth luxation, alveolar fracture, jaw fracture or luxation or fracture of the temporomandibular joint.

Is there any reaction in the teeth to cold and/or heat? A positive finding indicates exposure of dentin and therefore need for dentinal coverage.

Finally, a short **medical history** should reveal possible allergies, blood diseases and other information which could influence treatment.

The clinical examination

The clinical examination should first include examination of soft tissue wounds. If present, the penetrating nature of these should be determined, with emphasis on the possible presence of foreign bodies embedded within these wounds. Thereafter, the hard dental tissues are examined for the presence of infractions and fractures. The diagnosis of *infractions* is facilitated by directing the light beam parallel to the labial surface of the injured tooth (Fig. 1.5).

CHAPTER 1

Fig. 1.4. **Previous injury, permanent dentition**
The patient has just suffered enamel fractures of the incisors. However, a dental injury 4 years earlier has resulted in pulp necrosis of both central incisors and pulp canal obliteration, arrested root formation and secondary pulp necrosis of the left lateral incisor.

In the case of *crown fractures* a supplemental *luxation* diagnosis is also necessary in evaluating long-term pulp survival. Pulp exposures should be detected and their size noted, as well as the vascularity of the pulp (whether there is fresh hemorrhage, cyanosis or ischemia). Detection of pinpoint perforations is facilitated by thorough cleansing of the fracture surface.

Mobility testing should determine the extent of loosening, especially in axial direction of individual teeth (an indication of a severed vascular supply) and mobility of groups of teeth (an indication of fracture of the alveolar process).

Percussion testing, with a finger in small children or the handle of a metal instrument, has two functions. Tenderness to percussion in an axial direction (i.e. from the incisal edge) will indicate damage to the periodontal ligament. Percussion of the labial surface will yield either a high or low percussion tone. A high, metallic percussion tone is an indication that the injured tooth is locked into bone (as in lateral luxation or intrusion). At the follow-up periods, this tone indicates ankylosis. This finding can be confirmed if a finger is placed on the oral surface of the tooth to be tested. It is possible to feel the tapping of the instrument in a tooth with a normal periodontal ligament (PDL). In the case of intrusion, lateral luxation or ankylosis, percussion cannot be felt through the tooth tested.

Fig. 1.5. **Diagnosing infractions**
When the light beam is directed parallel to the labial surface infractions become very prominent.

EXAMINATION OF THE TRAUMATIZED PATIENT, WOUND HEALING AND TREATMENT PRINCIPLES

Fig. 1.6. **Complete radiographic and photographic examination of an anterior trauma**
Note how the injuries appear different on different exposures. Photographic registration of the trauma allows exact measurement of tooth displacement at a later date as well as complete documentation of the extent of injury. This injury consisted of lateral luxation of the left central incisor. Note how the occlusal exposure is superior in showing lateral displacement.

Electrometric sensibility testing should be carried out if at all possible, as it gives important information about the neurovascular supply to the involved teeth. The most reliable response is obtained when the electrode is placed on the incisal edge or the most incisal aspect of enamel in the case of crown fractures. It should be noted that young teeth with incomplete root formation do not respond consistently to sensibility testing; but the response at the time of injury provides a baseline value for comparison at later follow-up examinations. Finally, sensibility testing in the primary dentition may yield inconclusive information due to lack of patient cooperation.

In Appendix 1, an example of the emergency records used at the University Hospital in Copenhagen is presented (see pages 173 to 176). Appendix 2 provides a sample of the clinical examination form used at the time of injury and at follow-up examinations (see page 177).

The radiographic examination

The clinical examination should now have determined the area of obvious or suspected injury; that is the area to be examined radiographically. In the presence of a *penetrating lip lesion*, a soft tissue radiograph is indicated in order to locate eventual foreign bodies. It should be noted that the orbicularis oris muscles close tightly around foreign bodies in the lip, making them impossible to palpate; they can only be identified radiographically. This is accomplished by placing a dental film between the lips and the dental arch and using 25% of the normal exposure time (see Chapter 11, p. 165).

An occlusal exposure of the traumatized anterior region gives an excellent view of most *lateral luxations, apical and mid-root root fractures* and *alveolar fractures* (Fig. 1.7). The standard periapical bisecting angle exposure of each traumatized tooth gives information about *cervical root fractures* as well as other tooth displacements. Thus, a radiographic examination comprising 1 occlusal exposure and 3 periapical bisecting angle exposures of the traumatized region will provide maximum information in determining the extent of trauma.

With the combined information from the clinical and radiographic examinations, diagnosis and treatment planning can then be carried out.

Finally, photographic registration of the trauma is recommended, as it offers an exact documentation of the extent of injury which can be used in later treatment planning, legal claims, or for clinical research.

In the following the examination, features of a typical trauma case resulting from a fall from a bicycle are shown (Fig. 1.7).

Fig. 1.7. Examination and treatment of a combined soft and hard tissue injury
An 8-year-old girl has had a fall with her bike. She hit the ground with the lower part of her face. There is displacement of the right central incisor and laceration of the gingiva.

Percussion test
This test is first carried out on non-traumatized teeth so that the patient fully understands the purpose of this test. In this case both horizontal and vertical percussion gave no sensitivity reaction; and the percussion tone was high and metallic, indicating that the displaced tooth was locked into the alveolus (lateral luxation injury).

EXAMINATION OF THE TRAUMATIZED PATIENT, WOUND HEALING AND TREATMENT PRINCIPLES

Mobility and sensibility testing

Mobility is tested in vertical as well as in horizontal direction. In this case the tooth was immobile. Sensibility testing is carried out on the incisal edge in order to get maximum stimulation of the pulp. In this case there was no response to pulp testing.

Radiographic examination

A complete examination is made including three bisecting angle radiographs and an occlusal exposure. Note how the occlusal exposure is optimal for showing the apical displacement.

Essentials

- Obtain standardized data from the patient.
- Clean the traumatized region.
- History: When, where and how did the injury occur?
- Unconsciousness? ammesia? headache? nausea? vomiting?
- Disturbance in the bite?
- Reaction to cold or heat?
- Previous dental injury?
- Any allergies or serious illnesses?

Clinical examination

- Soft tissues.
- Hard tissues (enamel fracture, dentin or pulp exposures)?
- Abnormal mobility, tooth displacement.
- Tenderness to percussion, percussion (ankylosis) tone.
- Electrometric pulpal sensibility.

Radiographic examination

- Soft tissues.
- Occlusal radiographic exposure of the traumatized region.
- Periapical bisecting angle exposure of each traumatized tooth.

Final diagnosis and treatment planning

CHAPTER 1

Wound healing and
treatment principles

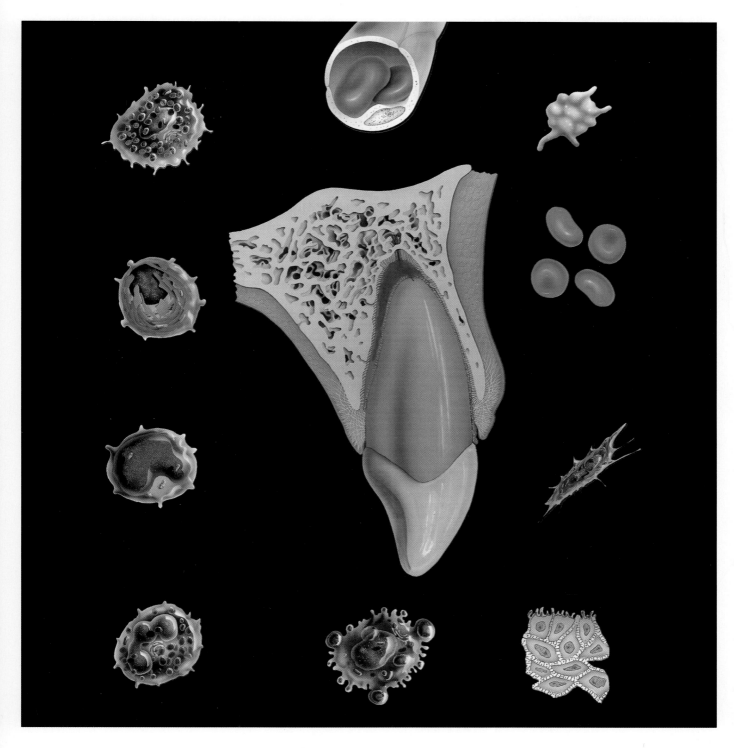

EXAMINATION OF THE TRAUMATIZED PATIENT, WOUND HEALING AND TREATMENT PRINCIPLES

Fig. 1.8. **Separation injury in the periodontal ligament.**

Fig. 1.9. **Crushing injury in the periodontal ligament.**

Fig. 1.10. **Wound healing module.** m = macrophages, f = fibroblasts, e = endothelial cells

Pattern of Injury

A traumatic dental injury represents acute transmission of energy to the tooth and supporting structures, which results in **fracture** and/or **displacement** of the tooth and/or **separation** or **crushing** of the supporting tissues (gingiva, periodontal ligament (PDL) and bone). In case of **separation** (e.g. extrusive luxation), the major part of the injury consists of cleavage of intercellular structures (collagen and intercellular substance), while there is limited damage to the cells in the area of trauma. This implies that wound healing can arise from existing cellular systems with a minimum of delay (Fig. 1.8).

In contrast, in a **crushing injury** (e.g. intrusive luxation), there is extensive damage to both cellular and intercellular systems; and damaged tissue must be removed by marcrophages and/or osteoclasts before the traumatized tissue can be restored. Such damage adds several weeks to the healing process and is reflected in the splinting period (Fig. 1.9).

Wound healing events

Wound healing events comprise revascularisation of ischemic tissue or formation of new tissue in case of tissue loss (Fig. 1.10). In both instances, wound healing takes place by a coordinated movement of cells into the traumatized area, where macrophages (m) form the healing front, followed by endothelial cells (e) and fibroblasts (f). Vascular loops are formed in a stroma of tissue dominated by immature collagen and proliferating fibroblasts. These cells are synchronized via chemical signals released by the involved cells and the surrounding tissue. This phenomenon has been termed the **wound healing module** (Fig. 1.10). This process appears to advance in the pulp and periodontum with a speed of approximately 0.5 mm a day.

In the following, wound healing responses will be described a as they appear in the case of **simple luxation injuries**, with only **separation injuries** of the PDL and the pulp, and **complicated luxation injuries** with **crushing injuries**.

Separation injury

PDL: After 1 week new collagen formation starts to unite the severed PDL fibres and results in initial consolidation of a luxated or a replanted tooth. After 2 weeks, repair of the principal fibers is so advanced that approximately two-thirds of the mechanical strength of the PDL has been regained.

Pulp: In luxated teeth with a severed vascular supply, ingrowth of new vessels into the pulp starts 4 days after injury and proceeds with a speed of approximately 0.5 mm per day in teeth with open apices. Revascularization is markedly influenced by

Fig. 1.11. **Repositioning after extrusion.**

Fig. 1.12. **Repositioning after lateral luxation.**

Fig. 1.13. **Orthodontic repositioning after intrusion.**

the size of the pulp-periodontal interface, being complete and predictable in teeth with open apices (≥ 1.0 mm) and rare in teeth with a narrow apical foramen (< 0.5 mm).

Crushing injury: In **complicated luxation injuries** with **crushing or other damage** of the PDL (e.g. desiccation after avulsion) complicating sequelae may occur which result in root resorption. These processes occur due to the loss of the protecting cementoblast layer and the epithelial rests of Mallassez along the root surface due to the traumatic events. When these cell layers disappear, there is free access of osteoclasts and macrophages to remove damaged PDL and cementum on the root surface which leads to root resorption. These processes are further described in Chapter 8.

Treatment effects on healing

Effects of repositioning: According to the force necessary to perform the repositioning procedure, more or less extra trauma will be transmitted to the periodontium and the pulp. This negative effect should be assessed in the light of possible benefits in subsequent wound healing of the approximation of wound surfaces. Thus, before repositioning a displaced tooth, one should evaluate how this might influence pulpal and periodontal healing, as well as the need for repositioning with respect to occlusion and esthetics. In the following, a outline is presented of the known effect of repositioning upon pulp and periodontal wound healing.

PDL: Incomplete – in contrast to complete – repositioning leads to a slight delay (approximately 2 weeks) in wound healing. However, the end result for the PDL is the same. If a part of the root surface is exposed to saliva (e.g. **extrusive luxation**), a loss of attachment in that particular region will occur unless complete repositioning is performed (Fig. 1.11). In **lateral luxation**, the value of repositioning is now known (Fig. 1.12).

Especially in those cases where forceful repositioning is necessary, spontaneous readjustment (in young individuals) or orthodontic readjustment should be considered. Occlusal and/or esthetic demands, however require immediate repositioning even in these cases.

After **intrusion** of permanent teeth, spontaneous re-eruption can usually only be expected in teeth with incomplete root formation (Fig. 1.13). In teeth with complete root formation, orthodontic re-eruption is possibly to be preferred over immediate repositioning in order to enhance marginal bone healing. However, there is no definite information yet available concerning this issue.

Pulp: Optimal repositioning leads to more rapid and more predictable pulpal revascularisation. Furthermore, if root formation is not complete, there is a good chance of survival of the epithelial root sheath and thereby and optimal chance of continued root growth.

19

Fig. 1.14. **Effect of splinting**

Fig. 1.15. **Effect of antibiotics**

Effects of splinting

PDL: In case of simple rupture of the PDL (e.g. **extrusive luxation**), rigid splinting does not promote healing. Flexible splinting is presently assumed to assist periodontal healing (Fig. 1.14). In situations with massive PDL cell death (e.g. **avulsion**), prolonged rigid splinting apparently leads to maintenance of initially formed ankylosis sites along the root surface. In these cases, short term semi-rigid splinting (i.e. 1 week to permit initial endodontics) appears to be the treatment of choice.

Pulp: Rigid splinting appears to slow down pulpal revascularization. Non-splinting, or flexible splinting is to be preferred.

Effects of antibiotics

PDL: Under experimental conditions, antibiotics administered either topically for 5 minutes before replantation of teeth in monkeys or systematically on the day of replantation have been found to decrease external root resorption. The explanation is most likely the killing of bacteria on the root surface which must otherwise be eliminated by an inflammatory response, possibly leading to an osteoclastic attack on the root surface (see p. 116).

Pulp: Systemic administration of antibiotics after luxation or root fractures, has not in clinical studies been found to enhance pulpal healing; nor could any effect be seen experimentally after replantaztion of extracted teeth in monkeys. In monkeys a 5-minute topical application of antibiotics was found to increase revascularization after replantation of extracted teeth with immature root formation.

Essentials

A traumatic dental injury represents acute transmission or energy to the tooth and supporting structures, which results in **fracture** and/or **displacement** of the tooth and/or **separation** or **crushing** of the supporting tissues (gingiva, periodontal ligament and bone).

The major part of a **separation injury** consists of cleavage of intercellular structures.

In a **crushing injury** there is extensive damage to both cellular and intercellular systems.

In case of a **separation injury** to the PDL initial consolidation is seen after 2 weeks.

In case of a **separation injury** to the pulp revascularisation occurs with a speed of 0.5 mm per day.

Complete repositioning of displaced teeth may enhance periodontal and pulpal healing.

Flexible splinting appears to promote healing in comparison to rigid splinting.

In root open teeth systemic antibiotics appears to decrease the risk of root resorption and possibly enhance pulpal revascularization.

CHAPTER 1

Crown fracture

CROWN FRACTURE

Fig. 2.1. **A frontal impact results in a crown fracture**

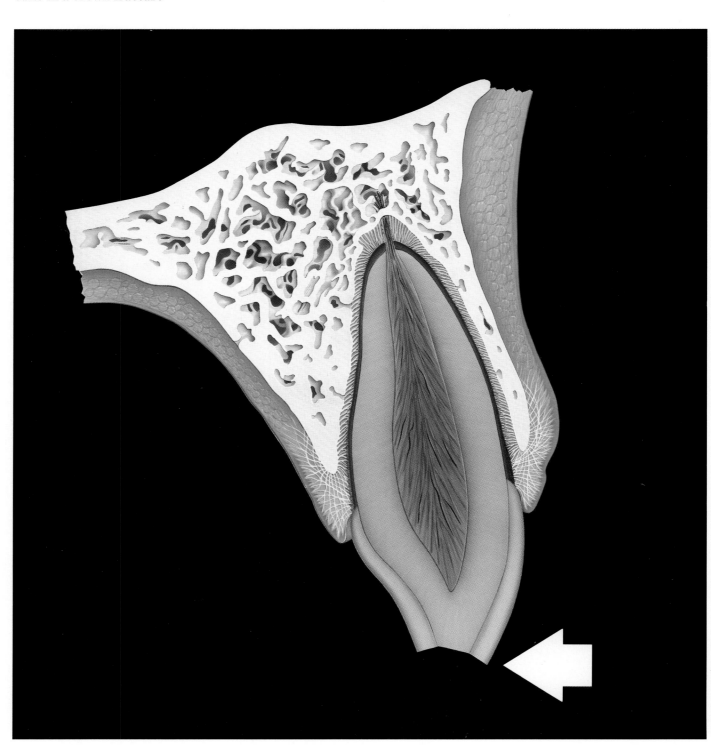

Pattern of injury and diagnosis

Crown fractures comprise the most frequent injuries in the permanent dentition. Apart from the loss of hard tissue, this injury can represent a hazard to the pulp. The usual cause of a crown fracture is a frontal impact, the energy of which exceeds the shear strength of enamel and dentin (Fig. 2.1). The tooth is thereby fractured in a horizontal pattern, following the course of the enamel rods. If the impact is from another direction, other lines of fracture may be seen. Pulpal status following crown fracture depends upon various factors: whether there is a concomitant luxation injury and the stage of root development, whether dentin has been exposed and, if so, whether dentinal coverage has been carried out.

Recent long-term clinical studies have shown that luxation injury concomitant to crown fractures with-or without pulp exposure is the primary source of pulpal complications following inju-

Fig. 2.2. Treatment of enamel fracture
Symmetry is reestablished by selective grinding of the injured and adjacent incisor.

CROWN FRACTURE

ry. Thus, even if exposed, but with an intact vascular supply, immunological defense systems in the pulp will combat bacterial invasion. However, with a luxation injury, vascularity is compromised or eliminated and bacterial invasion inevitable. (See Figs. 2.14 and 2.15).

In case of a pulp exposure, the following events take place. Soon after injury, the exposed pulp is covered with a layer of fibrin. A zone of acute inflammation is seen immediately subjacent to the exposure site. After 2 days, proliferative changes take place, whereby the pulp ultimately protrudes through the exposure. A significant finding is that the inflammatory zone is still confined to the most superficial 1-2 mm of the pulp even 1 week after injury. In case of an associated luxation injury, these events may be modified by total ischemia and autolysis of the pulp.

Fig. 2.3. **Treatment of an uncomplicated crown fracture with composite resin and the acid-etch technique**

CHAPTER 2

Treatment

In some cases of *enamel fractures*, selective grinding of the incisal edge is sufficient. In other cases, restoration with composite and the acid-etch technique is indicated. The extent and location of the fracture dictates the choice of treatment (Fig. 2.2).

On the other hand, *fractures of enamel and dentin* always require restoration in order to seal dentinal tubules and to restore esthetics. Restoration of esthetics can be achieved by composite resin build-up (Figs. 2.3 and 2.4), reattachment of the crown fragment using a dentin bonding agent, or by porcelain veneers or crowns.

At the time of injury, various factors can influence the choice of treatment as well as whether or not immediate definitive treatment can be performed. In many situations, a temporary restoration may be indicated. These include pulpal involvement, concomitant luxation injuries and lack of patient cooperation. Temporary restoration can be in the form of a pre-formed stainless steel or resin crown or temporary build-up using a temporary crown and bridge material or glass ionomer cement. If preformed crowns are to be cemented in place, it should be remembered that, in the case of concomitant luxation injuries, the periodontal ligament has been ruptured. In these cases, care must be taken to avoid forcing the temporary luting agent into the injured periodontal ligament space.

With respect to maintaining pulpal vitality, successful restoration of enamel-dentin crown fractures requires a hermetic seal of exposed dentinal tubules. This can be achieved by using glass ionomer cement, zinc oxide eugenol cement, hard setting calcium hydroxide paste or a dentin bonding agent (see later). While zinc oxide-eugenol cement has been found to be one of the best agents for producing a hermetic antibacterial seal, it is generally not recommended where a composite resin restoration is to be placed, as the eugenol component may interfere with polymerization at least with some composites. A similar effect has recently been seen with Dycal®, a hard setting calcium hydroxide paste where its use was found to halve bond strength of dental bonding agents. Therefore, in fractures with dentin exposure only, a dental bonding agent followed by a composite restoration is recommended. With pulp exposure, calcium hydroxide directly over the exposure, sealed in place with a glass ionomer cement, followed by a dentin bonding agent and composite is to be preferred.

Composite resin build-up (Fig. 2.4)

Preparation

Preparation of teeth for composite build-up has long been a subject of debate. It has been found that a *chamfer margin* (in contrast to a bevel) yields the best final result due to ease of finishing and the greater bulk of material at the final margin. The best restorative result is achieved if a rubber dam is used.

Fig. 2.4. Treatment of uncomplicated crown fracture with composite resin and acid-etch technique
Uncomplicated crown fracture in a 19-year-old girl.

Shade selection
Shade selection should be made *after* polishing with pure pumice and water and *before* application of the rubber dam, as the dehydrated enamel will change color.

Application of a rubber dam
A rubber dam is applied. Adjacent teeth should be included.

Chamfer preparation
A chamfer preparation is made labially and lingually, extending 2 mm from the fracture surface.

Etching enamel
The enamel is etched and a temporary crown form adapted.

Polymerization of composite
After curing, the surface anatomy is defined with a finishing diamond, whereas the general polishing is made with discs.

Finished restoration
Clinical and radiographic appearance of the restoration.

27

CROWN FRACTURE

Dentinal coverage/dental bonding

Bacterial invasion, especially in the presence of compromised pulpal vascularity, is the greatest threat to pulp vitality. A hermetic seal of dentinal tubules can be achieved using a bonding agent, which bonds to enamel and dentin simultaneously.

Acid etching

In order to ensure a tight seal against microleakage following restoration, adequate acid etching is required. That is, 30 seconds' etch followed by rinsing of the etched enamel surface with a copious flow of water for 20 seconds in order to remove all traces of etchant. Thereafter air drying to yield the characteristic mat enamel surface.

Choice of composite material

Light-cured resins have been found to possess the best color stability when compared with two-component self-cured resins. Crown fractures can be restored either using a layer build-up technique or by the use of standardized crown forms which are filled with the restorative material to be used. The choice of either technique is a personal one. However, it should be noted that light from the polymerizing lamp only penetrates approximately 2.0 mm and that in larger restorations adequate polymerization requires greater light exposure to achieve optimal material properties.

Reattachment of the crown fragment (Fig. 2.5)

This form of treatment has been shown to yield good esthetic results in that original tooth anatomy is restored with a material that abrades at a rate identical to that of the adjacent tooth substance and at the same time permits continual monitoring of pulpal status through the fragment.

Clinical procedure (Fig. 2.6)

The enamel-dentin fragment can either be brought to the dental clinic at the time of injury or can be recovered later. All fragments should be stored in either physiologic saline or tap water until bonding to prevent discoloration and/or infractions due to dehydration.

Fig. 2.5. **Reattachment of crown fragment using a dental bonding agent**

In the case of *uncomplicated* or *complicated fractures* and no concomitant luxation injury, bonding can be performed immediately. In the case of concomitant luxation injury with tooth displacement, a period of temporary restoration, corresponding to the splinting period after luxation must be included in the treatment schedule.

Temporization

In *uncomplicated fractures*, the exposed fracture surface (enamel and dentin) is disinfected and then covered with a glass ionomer cement).

In *complicated fractures*, pure calcium hydroxide (e.g. Calasept®) is placed over the exposure. The enamel and dentin of the fracture surface are then covered with glass ionomer cement. In both cases, the teeth are temporarily restored.

In the case of *concomitant luxation injuries*, the fixation period is the same as for the given trauma entity. The temporary restoration should stabilize the fractured tooth in order to avoid migration of the injured incisor or its antagonists.

Bonding of crown fractures

The bonding procedure for an uncomplicated crown fracture is illustrated in Fig. 2.6.

In the case of a complicated fracture, pulpal considerations are discussed later. Bonding is either carried out at the time of pulp capping or pulpotomy In the case of concomitant luxations, bonding can be performed when the splint and temporary restoration is removed. At that time, the temporary restoration is removed.

All soft tissue remnants from the exposure site are removed. The fracture surface is disinfected and the barrier covered with bonded composite or glass ionomer cement. Pulpal remnants in the crown fragment are removed with a round bur.

If necessary, the fragment is further hollowed out to accommodate the dressing over the hard tissue barrier and thus allow optimal repositioning of the fragment. Thereafter, bonding is performed as for uncomplicated fractures.

After bonding, patients may use the teeth normally. Limitations in use, however, include all horizontal occlusal forces, e.g. pulling on chewy foods (hard breads, tough meats, toffees).

Fig. 2.6. **Treatment of an uncomplicated crown fracture by reattaching the crown fragment with a dental bonding agent and reinforcement of the bonding site with composite resin and the acid-etch technique**
This 10-year-old boy has fractured his central incisor after a fall from his skateboard. The fracture is close to the mesial pulp horn.

Testing pulpal sensibility
Pulpal response to sensibility testing is normal. The radiographic examination shows no displacement or root fracture.

Testing the fit of the fragment

The fragment fits exactly. The enamel surface is intact, with no apparent defect at the enamel margins.

Etching enamel

The fragment is fastened to a piece of sticky wax for the ease of handling.

Enamel on both fracture surfaces as well as a 2-mm wide collar of enamel cervical and incisal to the fracture are etched for 30 seconds with 35% phosphoric acid gel, being sure that the etchant does not come in contact with dentin.

Removal of the etchant

The fracture surfaces are rinsed thoroughly with a copious flow of water for 20 seconds.

Drying the fracture surfaces

The fracture surfaces are air dried for 10 seconds. NOTE: To avoid entrapment of air in the dentinal tubules and a subsequent chalky mat discoloration of the fragment, the ait stream must be directed parallel with the fracture surface and not perpendicular to it.

32

Conditioning the dentin with EDTA and GLUMA®
The fracture surfaces are conditioned with EDTA for 20 seconds; followed by 10 seconds water rinse and 10 seconds air drying. Thereafter 20 seconds GLUMA® and 10 seconds air drying.

Bonding the fragment
The fracture surfaces are covered with a creamy mixture of a filled composite and its unfilled resin. After repositioning of the fragment, the composite is light-polymerized 60 seconds facially and 60 seconds orally.

Polymerization of the palatal aspect of the fracture

Removal of surplus composite
With a straight scalpel blade or composite finishing knive surplus composite is removed from the fracture site. The interproximal bonding area are finished with finishing strips.

CROWN FRACTURE

Reinforcing the fracture site.
A round diamond bur is used to create a "double chamfer" margin 1 mm coronally and apically to the fracture line. To achieve optimal esthetics, the chamfer follows an undulating path along the fracture line.

Finishing the labial surface
The labial aspect of the crown is restored with composite.

Reinforcing the palatal aspect of the fracture
The restoration is contoured using abrasive discs. The palatal aspect of the fracture is reinforced using the same procedure. Due to its position, esthetic consideration is less. The preparation can, therefore, follow the fracture line exactly.

The final restoration
The condition 1 month after reattachment of the crown fragment.

Complicated crown fractures – pulpal considerations

Treatment of *pulp exposures* depends upon pulpal healing potential and the desirability of maintaining a vital pulp. Thus profound crown fracture of a mature tooth might dictate pulpal extirpation to permit restoration with a post-retained crown (Fig. 2.7).

In the event that a vital pulp is desired (as in young individuals) the following conditions must be fulfilled: 1.) The pulp should have been free of inflammation prior to injury; and 2.) any associated injury to the PDL must not have compromised the vascular supply to the pulp (Fig. 2.8).

If these conditions can be met, pulp capping and partial pulpotomy are the treatments of choice (Figs. 2.9 and 2.10). The choice between these two treatment procedures is unclear at present. Therefore, only a few *unsupported* guidelines can be given. Thus, pulp capping should be used primarily for small exposures soon after injury (possibly within the first 24 hours) and where a restoration can be placed which provides a tight seal against bacterial invasion (Figs. 2.9 and 2.11).

In larger exposures with longer post-trauma intervals, a partial pulpotomy should be performed to a depth of 2 mm (Figs. 2.12 to 2.13). Later direct monitoring of the hard tissue barrier is not recommended, at this implies risk of renewed exposure to bacte-

Fig. 2.7. **Treatment of a complicated crown fracture by pulpal extirpation**

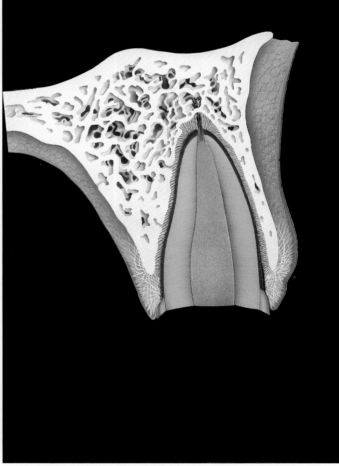

Fig. 2.8. Evaluation of pulpal integrity following crown fracture
The right central incisor was slightly loosened but not displaced at the time of injury (subluxation). The left central incisor was tender to percussion (concussion). The cyanotic, exposed pulp of the subluxated incisor reflects a compromised circulation following trauma. The exposed pulp of the left central incisor reflects intact circulation.

ria. Therefore, the amputation site should either be covered with hard setting calcium hydroxide cement followed by a thin layer of glass ionomes cement or MTA® and the tooth restored using a dental adhesive to ensure a bacteria-tight seal.

Fig. 2.9. Treatment of a complicated crown fracture by pulp capping

Three months after injury, the exposure site is uncovered. The amputation material as well as the necrotic pulp tissue immediately above the hard tissue barrier are removed. If the barrier appears intact, a bacteria-tight material is placed (e.g. glass ionomer cement or a dentin-bonded composite). The tooth can then be restored either with conventional composite build-up using the acid-etch technique or bonding of the original crown fragment using a dentin bonding system. The need for a hermetic seal seems relevant (although not proven), as all hard tissue barriers contain numerous vascular inclusions which may allow bacterial invasion of the pulp.

Figs. 2.11-2.13 illustrate treatment of different types of crown fractures.

Fig. 2.10. **Treatment of a complicated crown fracture by partial pulpotomy**

CROWN FRACTURE

Follow-up procedures

Crown fractured teeth should be followed in order to diagnose pulpal complications. A useful follow-up schedule is 1 and 2 months and 1 year after injury. Signs of pulp necrosis include loss of pulpal sensibility, coronal discoloration, periapical radiolucency and persistent tenderness to percussion. However, none of these signs is pathognomonic.

Fig. 2.11. Treatment of a complicated crown fracture by pulp capping and a composite resin restoration
This 12-year-old boy has suffered a crown fracture with a small pulp exposure.

Pulp capping
After isolation with a rubber dam, the pulp exposure is covered with a calcium hydroxide paste (e.g. Calasept®). The remaining dentin is covered with a hard-setting calcium hydroxide cement, whereafter the tooth is restored with a composite. (Courtesy of Dr. M. Cvek, Eastman Dental Institute, Stockholm).

Fig. 2.12. Treatment of a complicated crown fracture by pulpotomy and subsequent bonding of the crown fragment
This 9-year-old boy has suffered a dental trauma 1 day previously. Note the good vascularity of the exposed pulp.

Pulpotomy
The tooth is isolated with a rubber dam and a pulpotomy is carried out using calcium hydroxide (i.e. Calasept®) and a glass ionomer cement as a cover.

Testing the fit of the fragment
The fragment is tried in to ensure that the cover over the pulpotomy does not prevent correct repositioning of the fragment.

Bonding the fragment
The clinical and radiographic condition is shown 4 years after bonding. (Courtesy of Dr. M. Cvek, Eastman Dental Institute, Stockholm).

Fig. 2.13. Complicated crown fracture treated by pulpotomy and composite restoration

A 10-year-old boy who has suffered a crown fracture 2 days previously.

Clinical condition

A large pulp exposure is found.

Isolation with a rubber dam

After administration of an infiltration anesthesia, the tooth is isolated with a rubber dam. An inverted diamond cone is used for the pulpotomy.

Pulpotomy

The pulpotomy is carried out to a depth of 2.0 mm, using a copious water spray from the airrotor, supplemented with an extra saline spray from a syringe.

Preparing the cavity
The access cavity to the pulpotomy site should be boxlike,
with a slight undercut in dentin.

Applying the amputation material
Hemostasis is awaited. After
some minutes, this will usually
occur. Otherwise, slight pressure
applied with a cotton pellet
soaked in a anesthetic solution
with vasoconstrictor or calcium
hydroxide can be used. After
complete arrest of bleeding. calcium hydroxide paste (e.g. Cala-
sept®) is placed on the pulpal
wound.

Compressing the amputation material
The material is compressed
slightly using a cotton pellet.
Thereafter, the entry site is
covered with hard-setting calcium hydroxide cement.

Restoration
The tooth has been restored
using a composite resin and a
dentin bonding agent. (Courtesy
of Dr. M. Cvek, Eastman Dental
Institute, Stockholm).

CROWN FRACTURE

General prognosis

The prognosis of crown fractures appears to depend primarily upon the presence of associated periodontal ligament injury and secondarily upon the extent of dentin exposed and the age of the pulp exposure (see Figs. 2.14 to 2.17).

Fig. 2.14. **Pulpal healing after uncomplicated crown fractures in teeth with open apices according to type of luxation injury** (after Andreasen & Andreasen 1989).

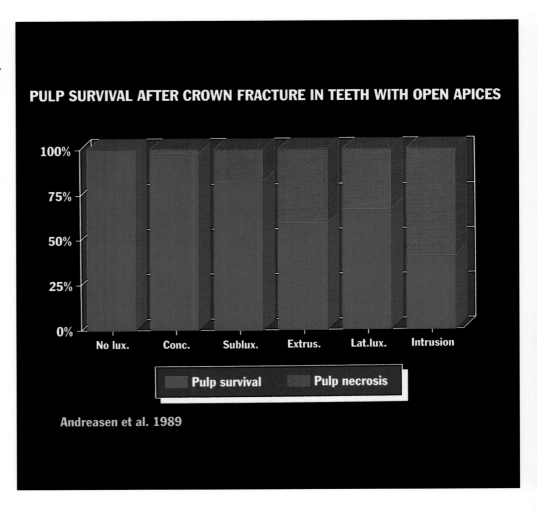

Fig. 2.15. **Pulpal healing after uncomplicated crown fractures in teeth with closed apices according to type of luxation injury** (after Andreasen & Andreasen 1989).

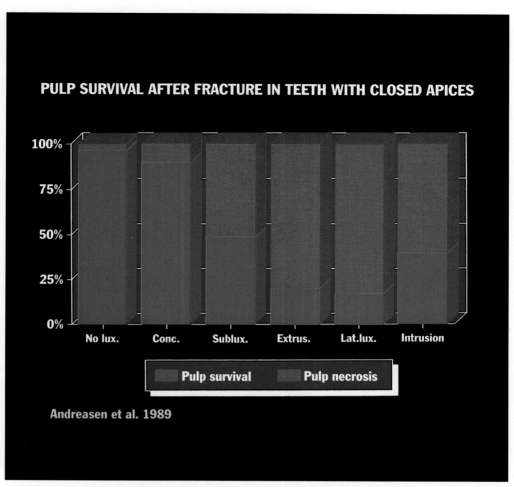

Fig. 2.16. **Pulpal healing after pulp capping** (after Ravn 1982).

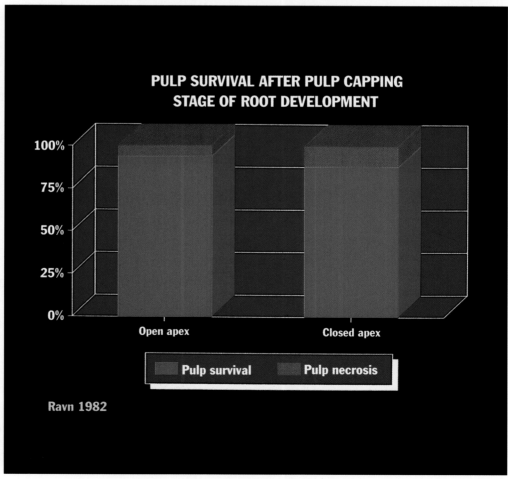

CROWN FRACTURE

Fig. 2.17. **Pulpal healing after partial pulpotomy** (after Cvek 1993).

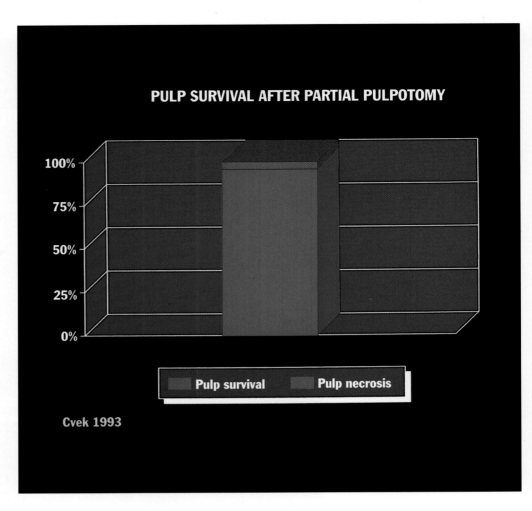

PULP SURVIVAL AFTER PARTIAL PULPOTOMY

Pulp survival   Pulp necrosis

Cvek 1993

Essentials

Crown fractures represent a hazard to the pulp only if the following has occurred:
– Associated periodontal ligament injury.

Treatment principles of crown fractures imply the following:
Fractures of enamel, depending on the site and extent of fracture:
– Selective grinding of the incisal edge and possibly of the adjacent tooth to reestablish symmetry.
– Acid-etch composite restoration.

Fractures of enamel and dentin
A bacteria-tight cover of the exposed dentin should be established as soon after injury as possible. Dentinal coverage can include dentin bonded composites, glass ionomer cements or bonding of a crown fragment. Lately veneers have succesfully been used to restore crown fractured teeth.

Pulp exposures
The exposed pulp can usually be treated successfully (i.e. by the formation of a calcified bridge) under the following circumstances:

- No inflammation prior to trauma.
- Intact vascular supply after trauma.

Two treatment options exist:
- Pulp capping.
- Partial pulpotomy.

Which of these two treatment procedures is to be preferred has not yet been determined; however, the following conditions appear to favor *pulpotomy* rather than pulp capping:
- Long exposure period after trauma (i.e. more than 24 h).
- Large exposures (limit not established).
- Reduced vascularity due to a concomitant luxation injury.

Treatment procedures: *Pulp capping*
- Isolate the pulp exposure.
- Cover the pulp with a calcium hydroxide material (either hard-setting cement or pure calcium hydroxide paste).
- Restore the tooth immediately with a bacteria-tight restoration. Later assessment of the hard tissue barrier implies risk of renewed exposure to bacteria. Thereafter, the hard tissue barrier is re-covered with glass ionomer cement or a composite resin retained with a dental bonding agent; and thereafter the tooth can be restored.

Treatment procedures: *Pulpotomy*
- Isolate the pulp exposure.
- Amputate the pulp to a level approximately 2 mm below the exposure site, or to where fresh bleeding is seen.
- If *immediate restoration* is desired, cover the exposure with a hard-setting calcium hydroxide cement (e.g. Dycal® or Life®).
- If *later assessment of the hard tissue barrier* is desired, cover the exposure with pure calcium hydroxide paste, cover the entire fracture surface (enamel and dentin) with a hard-setting calcium hydroxide cement and a temporary restoration for a period of 3 months. At that time, uncover the amputation site, remove the necrotic pulp tissue immediately above the hard tissue barrier and restore with a bacteria-tight restoration.

45

CHAPTER 3

Crown-root fracture

Fig. 3.1. **Fracture mechanism in a crown–root fracture**
The horizontal impact produces compression zones at the point of impact cervically on the palatal aspect and apically on the labial aspect of the root. The shearing stress zones which extend between the compression zones determine the course of the fracture.

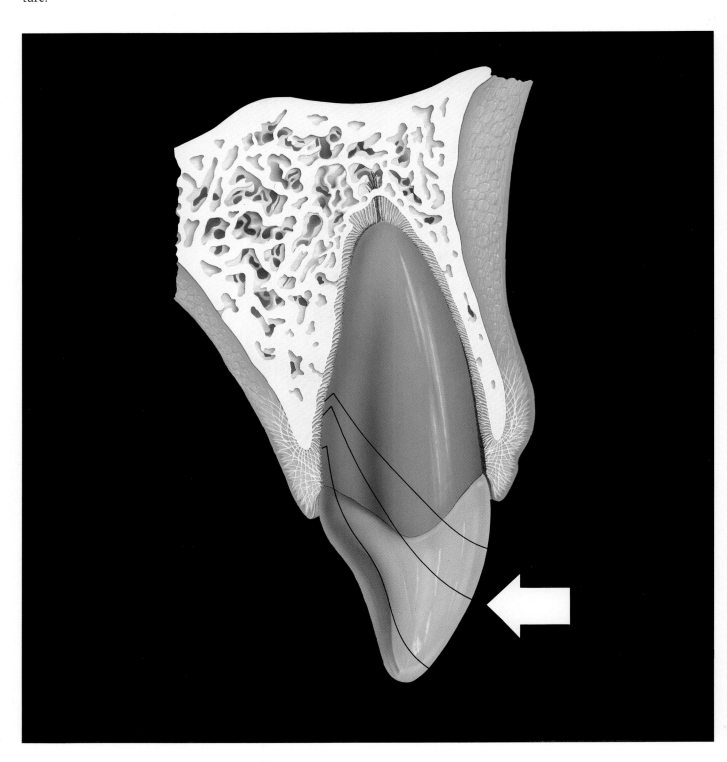

Pattern of injury and diagnosis

This trauma entity is quite common and usually presents serious treatment problems due to the complex nature of the injury. Most of these fractures occur as the result of a horizontal impact. If the force of the impact exceeds the shearing strength of the hard dental tissues, a fracture will occur which initially follows the enamel rods of the labial surface of the crown and then takes an oblique course below the palatal gingival crest (Fig. 3.1). During its course through dentin, the fracture will often expose the pulp. The fracture line is usually single; but multiple fractures can occur, often commencing from the depth of the primary fracture.

A crown-root fracture left untreated usually results in pain from mastication due to movement of the coronal fragment; but is otherwise without symptoms.

The pathological events in case of no treatment comprise inflammatory changes in the pulp, periodontal ligament and the gingiva due to plaque accumulation in the line of fracture (Fig. 3.2).

The *clinical diagnosis* of a crown-root fracture is apparent when the coronal fragment is mobile (Fig. 3.2). The *radiographic diagnosis* is more difficult, at least with respect to its lingual extent, as the fracture line is usually perpendicular to the central radiographic beam (Fig. 3.2).

Fig. 3.2. **Clinical and radiographic diagnosis of a crown-root fracture**
The coronal fragment is mobile. The radiographs are not able to reveal the apical limit of the fracture.

CROWN-ROOT FRACTURE

Treatment

Most crown-root fractured teeth can be saved. In the following, various treatment procedures will be shown, including treatment indications, treatment principles and a cost-benefit analysis of their use.

Treatment at the time of injury

Definitive treatment of a crown-root fracture can be complicated and time-consuming – not a treatment to be started in the midst of a busy schedule or late at night.

The primary goal at the initial visit is, therefore, elimination of pain, primarily due to mobility of the coronal fragment.

This is easily achieved by splinting the mobile fragment to adjacent teeth using acid etch and temporary crown and bridge resin or glass ionomer cement. Once this is done, the patient can be dismissed, to return at a later date for definitive therapy. At the initial visit, pulpal therapy is usually not indicated, as pulpal vascularity apical to the fracture line is usually intact and capable of combating infection.

Fig. 3.3. **Removal of the coronal fragment and supragingival restoration**

Removal of the coronal fragment with subsequent restoration above gingival level

Treatment principle. To allow the subgingival portion of the fracture to heal (presumably with formation of a long junctional epithelium), whereafter the coronal portion can be restored either by: bonding the original tooth fragment where the subgingival portion of the fragment has been removed using a dentin bonding system, a composite build-up using dentin and enamel bonding systems, or a crown restoration (Figs. 3.3 and 3.4).

Fig. 3.4. Removal of the coronal fragment and supragingival restoration
This 16-year-old girl has suffered a crown-root fracture which has exposed the palatal root surface. The clinical condition is shown after gingivectomy.

Condition 1 week after gingivectomy
The palatal fragment has been removed and the exposed root dentin smoothed with a bur; the exposed dentin covered with calcium hydroxide and a temporary crown. Two weeks later creeping reattachment is seen and the palatal of the crown restored with a dentin bonded composite resin restoration.

Follow-up
Clinical and radiographic condition 4 years after treatment. (Courtesy of Dr. B. Malmgren, Eastman Institute, Stockholm, Sweden)

CROWN-ROOT FRACTURE

Indication. This procedure should be limited to superficial fractures that do not involve the pulp.

Treatment procedure. The loose fragment is removed as soon as possible after injury. Rough edges along the fracture surface below the gingiva may be smoothed with a chisel. The remaining crown is covered with a temporary crown whose margin ends supragingivally. Once gingival healing is seen (after 2-3 weeks), the crown can be restored.

Cost-benefit. The method is easily followed and treatment time is short. However, the long-term effect with respect to the pulp and periodontium remains to be documented.

Removal of the coronal fragment supplemented by gingivectomy and osteotomy and subsequent restoration with a post-retained crown

Treatment principle. To convert the subgingival fracture to a supragingival fracture with the help of gingivectomy and osteotomy (Fig. 3.5).

Indication. Should only be used where the surgical technique does not compromise the esthetic result, i.e. only the palatal aspect of the fracture must be exposed in this manner.

Treatment procedure. The coronal fragment is removed and a gingivectomy and osteotomy are performed. Bone is removed 2 mm below the level of the fracture (Fig. 3.5). At the same time, the pulp is extirpated. The root filling can be placed at the same session or at a later appointment. Once the root filling is complete, an impression is taken for a post-retained crown. A potential threat to tooth survival following crown-root fracture and subsequent restoration with a post-core-support crown is the risk of subsequent fractures eminating from the root canal. A possible method to prevent these cracks is the use of a dental bonding agent and a resin composite luting agent for post-core cementation.

Cost-benefit. Treatment time is short. However, long-term follow-up of these restorations has shown a slight tendency for the crowns to migrate labially. Furthermore, the palatal gingiva was often hyperplastic and inflamed despite good adaptation of the crown margins.

Removal of the coronal fragment and surgical extrusion of the root

Treatment principle. To surgically move the fracture to a supragingival position (Fig. 3.6).

Indication. Should only be used where the root portion is long enough to accommodate a post-retained crown.

Treatment. As soon after injury as possible, the coronal frag-

Fig. 3.5. Removal of the coronal fragment and surgical exposure of the fracture
Clinical and radiographic appearance of a complicated crown-root fracture.

Exposing the fracture site
The coronal fragment is removed. A combined gingivectomy and osteotomy expose the fracture surface.

Constructing a post-retained crown
After taking an impression, a post-retained full crown is fabricated.

The finished restoration
The clinical and radiographic condition 2 months after insertion of the crown.

53

CROWN-ROOT FRACTURE

ment is removed (Fig. 3.7). The apical fragment is luxated with an elevator and removed with forceps. The pulp can be extirpated at this time. The root is then moved into a more coronal position and secured in that position with sutures and/or a splint. In case of palatally inclined fractures, 180° rotation can often imply that only slight extrusion is necessary to accommodate crown preparation. After 2-3 weeks, the tooth can be treated endodontically. After another 1-2 months, the tooth can be restored with a post-retained crown.

Cost–benefit. Several clinical studies have indicated that this is a safe and rapid method for the treatment of crown-root fractures. However, pulp vitality must be sacrificed.

Removal of the coronal fragment and subsequent orthodontic extrusion of the root

Treatment principle. To orthodontically move the fracture to a supragingival position (Fig. 3.8).

Indication. The same as for surgical extrusion, but is more time consuming.

Fig. 3.6. **Removal of the coronal fragment and surgical extrusion of the root**

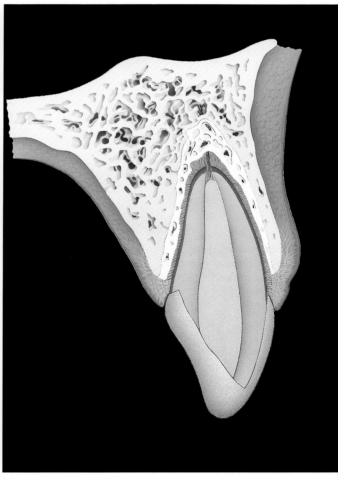

Fig. 3.7. Removal of the coronal fragment and surgical extrusion of the root

A complicated crown-root fracture in a 13-year-old boy.
The loose fragment is stabilized immediately after injury with a temporary crown and bridge material using the acid-etch technique.

Incision of the PDL

Using a specially contoured surgical blade, after administration of a local anesthetic.

Luxation of the root

The root is then luxated with a narrow elevator which is placed at the mesiopalatal and distopalatal corners respectively.

Extracting the root

The root is extracted and inspected for additional fractures.

CROWN-ROOT FRACTURE

Replanting the apical fragment

The root is tried in different positions in order to establish where the fracture is optimally exposed yet with minimal extrusion. In this instance, optimal repositioning was achieved by rotating the root 45°.

Stabilization of the apical fragment during healing

The root is splinted to adjacent teeth. The pulp is extirpated and the access cavity to the root canal closed.

Root filling

Two weeks after initial treatment, endodontic therapy can be continued, in the form of an interim dressing with calcium hydroxide. The root canal is obturated with gutta percha and sealer as far apically as possible 1 month after surgical extrusion.

Completion of the restoration

Two months after surgical extrusion, healing has occurred and it is possible to complete the restoration.

Treatment. The coronal fragment is removed, the pulp extirpated and the root canal filled (Fig. 3.9). Alternatively, the endodontic therapy can be performed prior to the removal of the coronal fragment (i.e. while the coronal fragment is temporarily splinted to the adjacent teeth). This might facilitate the endodontic procedure. Alternatively, a pulp capping or pulpotomy may be performed, a situation which is indicated if root formation is not complete (Fig. 3.10). Thereafter, orthodontic traction is applied to either a bracket fastened to the labial surface of the fragment or to a hook cemented into the root canal. The root is then extruded over a period of 2-3 weeks. The gingiva will follow the path of the extruding root, thus necessitating a gingivectomy once extrusion is complete. Moreover, incision of the circumferential periodontal fibers and fixation of the tooth for 14 days is necessary to prevent re-intrusion of the extruded incisor. The tooth is then retained for 3-4 weeks, whereafter it can be restored with a composite build-up or a post-retained crown.

Fig. 3.8. **Removal of the coronal fragment and orthodontic extrusion of the root**

CROWN-ROOT FRACTURE

Cost-benefit. The procedure is slow and cumbersome. However, it provides excellent esthetic results and the gingival health appears to be optimal. Pulp vitality can be saved if indicated (teeth with immature root formation).

Follow-up procedures

Each procedure bears with it routine monitoring of periodontal status clinically and radiographically. Follow-up intervals should be at 2 months after completed treatment and 1 year after injury.

General prognosis

See the individual treatment procedures.

Fig. 3.9. **Removal of the coronal fragment, pulp extirpation and orthodontic extrusion**
A complicated crown root fracture in a 13-year-old boy.

Endodontic treatment
The pulp has been extirpated. After a period with a calcium hydroxide interim dressing, the canal is filled with gutta percha and sealer.

Applying extrusion appliances
Two premolars and the canine are used as anchorage for the orthodontic appliances.

Orthodontic extrusion
The tooth is extruded quickly over a period of 2-3 weeks in order to prevent coronal migration of marginal bone.

Condition 1 year after extrusion
The root has been extruded and the dentin covered with glass ionomer cement and then restored with composite (Courtesy of Dr. B. Malmgren and E. Köndell, Eastman Dental Institute, Stockholm).

CROWN-ROOT FRACTURE

Fig. 3.10. Removal of the coronal fragment, pulpotomy and orthodontic extrusion

A complicated crown-root fracture of a mandibular central incisor in a 14-year-old girl.

Removing the loose fragment

The coronal fragment is removed, revealing a large pulp exposure. However, pulpal vascularity appears intact.

Pulpotomy

A pulpotomy is performed. The level of amputation is placed at the cervical area, and the tooth temporarily restored with glass ionomer cement.

Orthodontic extrusion

After verification of a hard tissue closure at the amputation site, the tooth is extruded using an orthodontic appliance.

Extrusion complete
After extrusion and a fibrotomy the tooth is retained using an acid-etch retainer employing glass fiber and composite resin.

Restoration completed
The tooth has been restored using a combination of glass ionomer cement and composite resin (Courtesy of Dr. B. Malmgren & K. Ridell, Eastman Dental Institute, Stockholm).

Essentials

Crown-root fractures may or may not involve the pulp.

Clinical diagnosis depends upon mobility of the coronal fragment. Radiographic diagnosis, however, is uncertain as it is usually impossible to determine the oral extent of fracture.

Emergency treatment

Stabilization of the coronal fragment by splinting to adjacent teeth.

Treatment principles include the following
- **Removal of the coronal fragment and supragingival restoration** (e.g. by bonding the original crown fragment after removing the subgingival portion, with composite build-up or a crown) in order to permit subgingival healing, presumably with a long junctional epithelium.
- **Removal of the coronal fragment supplemented by gingivectomy and/or osteotomy,** in order to convert the subgingival fracture surface to supragingival in situations where esthetics permit; thereafter, restoration (e.g. with a post-retained crown).
- **Removal of the coronal fragment and surgical or orthodontic extrusion of the root,** to move the fracture surface to a more optimal location for final restoration.

61

Root fracture

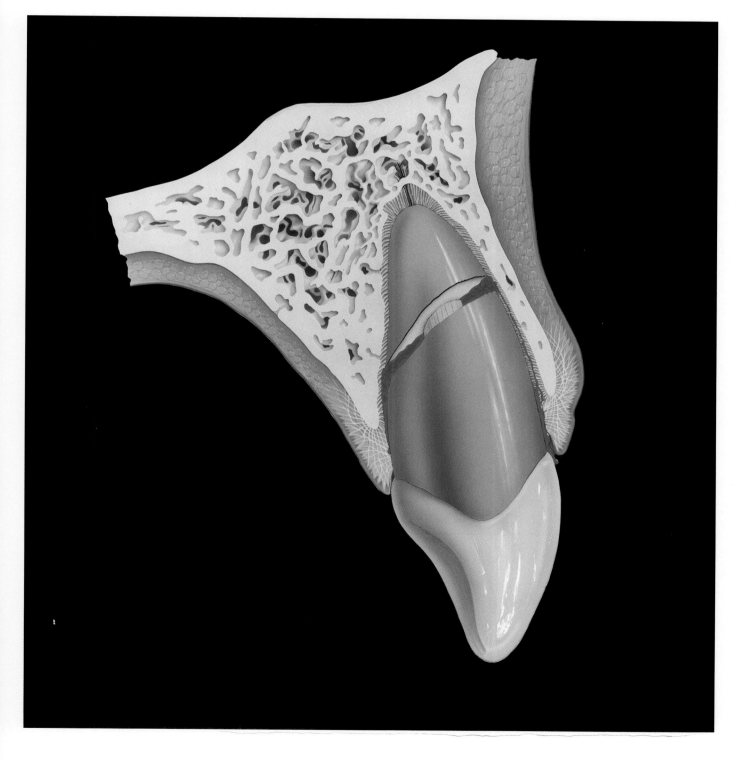

ROOT FRACTURE

Fig. 4.1. **Mechanism of root fracture**
A frontal impact displaces the tooth palatally and results in a root fracture and displacement of the coronal fragment. This leads to both pulp and PDL damage in the coronal fragment.

Pattern of injury and diagnosis

Root fractures are relatively uncommon injuries, but represent complex healing patterns due to concomitant injury to the pulp, periodontal ligament, dentin and cementum. The fracture usually results from a horizontal impact. Fractures in the apical- and middle-thirds of the root normally take an oblique course, being placed more apically on the labial aspect than on the palatal (Fig. 4.1). A rather steep radiographic exposure is needed for optimal fracture detection in these locations. However, as the level of fracture approaches the cervical one-third, the direction of fracture changes, being more or less perpendicular to the fractures in the apical- and middle-thirds. These fractures obviously require a different angulation of the central beam in order to be detected radiographically. Thus, more than one radiographic exposure is necessary to ensure detection of all root fractures.

The frontal impact tends to force the coronal fragment palatally and in a slightly extruded direction. In this way the pulp may be stretched, but may or may not be severed, due to its inherent elasticity.

The healing events which subsequently take place are primarily dependent upon two conditions: whether the pulp is severed and whether bacteria have invaded the fracture line. If the pulp is intact after injury, a dentin callus is formed between the two fragments after some weeks, whereafter the peripheral aspect of the

Fig. 4.2. Hard tissue healing after root fracture
The pulp is ruptured at the level of the fracture. Fracture healing with ingrowth of cells originating from the apical half of the pulp ensures hard tissue union of the fracture.

ROOT FRACTURE

65

Fig. 4.3. **Connective tissue healing after root fracture**
The pulp is ruptured or severely stretched at the level of the fracture. Healing is dominated by ingrowth of cells originating from the periodontal ligament and results in interposition of connective tissue between the two fragments.

Fig. 4.4. **Non-healing due to infection in the line of fracture**
Infection occurs in the avascular coronal aspect of the pulp. Granulation tissue is soon formed which originates from the periodontal ligament. Accumulation of cells between the two fragments causes separation of the fragments and loosening of the coronal fragment.

fracture is healed by cementum deposition, a process which can take place over a period of several years (Fig. 4.2).

If the pulp has been ruptured, revascularization of the coronal aspect of the pulp has to take place prior to fracture healing. The exact nature of this process is not yet known. But it is suspected that two events can take place; namely, invasion of cells derived from the apical pulp or invasion of cells from the periodontal ligament (Fig. 4.3). Depending upon the source of cells entering the coronal pulp canal, healing of the fracture will take place by either union with hard tissue or by interposition of connective tissue (from the periodontal ligament) respectively.

In the event that bacteria gain access to the coronal pulp in its avascular condition, healing of the pulp is impossible and an accumulation of granulation tissue between root fragments will result as a response to the infected coronal aspect of the pulp (Fig. 4.4).

Treatment

To facilitate pulpal and periodontal ligament healing, it is considered essential (although not proven) that a displaced coronal fragment be optimally repositioned. Furthermore, that splinting be maintained for a 3-weeks period where PDL healing normally has stabilized the tooth (Fig. 4.5). In Figs. 4.6 and 4.7, repositioning and splinting of root fractures with different types of displacement (luxation) of the coronal fragment are demonstrated.

Follow-up procedures

Sensibility testing and radiographic examination should be performed 3 weeks, 6 weeks and 6 months after injury (see Appendix 4, page 179).

Radiographic guidelines. Recent clinical studies have indicated that certain radiographic findings can be used as predictors for root fracture healing.

Resorption within the root canal originating at the fracture line is apparently a stage in healing following pulpal damage after trauma. This has been found to be followed by later mineralization events and healing by interposition of connective tissue. This condition does not require treatment, but does require regular follow-up control.

Resorption within bone at the level of the fracture line is, however, an indicator of pulp necrosis, usually of the coronal fragment. This condition requires endodontic therapy; that is, extirpation of the necrotic coronal pulp, interim dressing with a calcium hydroxide paste and finally gutta percha root filling. It should be noted that successful endodontic treatment will lead to healing with interposition of connective tissue.

Pulp canal obliteration of the coronal and apical root canals indicates a response to pulpal injury and subsequent healing by interposition of connective tissue between fragments.

General prognosis

Two major factors can predict prognosis for pulpal healing after root fracture: the stage of root development at the time of injury and dislocation of the coronal fragment. Figs. 4.8 and 4.9 show the risk of pulp necrosis as related to the stage of root development. Other complications, such as progressive root resorption and loss of marginal bone support are very rare.

It should be noted that, while healing by hard tissue union is optimal, interposition of connective tissue is also an acceptable healing entity. It is not presently known how the two forms of healing affect the life expectancy of root-fractured incisors.

Finally, location of the root fracture has not been shown to affect pulp survival after injury. Thus, in patients with good periodontal health, root fractures of the cervical third could be treated successfully by permanent interproximal fixation using the acid-etch technique.

Fig. 4.5. **Principles for treatment of root fractures**
Treatment of root fractures consists of complete repositioning and splinting, preferably with a passively applied splint (see text), until stabilization of healing in the PDL has taken place.

Fig. 4.6. **Treatment of a laterally luxated root fracture**
This 13-year-old boy received a horizontal blow to the left maxillary central incisor.

Clinical examination
The tooth reacts to sensibility testing, indicating an intact vascular supply. There is a high metallic sound elicited by the percussion test, indicating lateral luxation of the coronal fragment. The tooth is locked firmly in its displaced position, confirming the luxation diagnosis.

Repositioning
Because of the force necessary to reposition a laterally luxated tooth, regional block anesthesia is administered prior to repositioning. Firm pressure is applied to the facial bone plate at the fracture level in order to displace the coronal fragment out of its alveolar "lock." This is followed by horizontal (forward) pressure at the palatal aspect of the incisal edge, which repositions the coronal fragment into its original position.

Verifying repositioning
The correct position of the coronal fragment is confirmed radiographically.

Fixation procedure

The acid-etch technique and a temporary crown and bridge material is used. Phosphoric acid gel is applied for 30 seconds to the facial surfaces of the injured and adjacent non-injured teeth. The tooth surfaces are then rinsed thoroughly with a stream of water for 20-30 seconds and blown dry. A mat enamel surface indicates adequate etching.

Applying the splinting material

A temporary crown and bridge material (e.g. Protemp®) is applied to the etched enamel surfaces. The bulk of the material should be placed on the mesial and distal corners of the traumatized and the adjacent, non-injured incisors. After setting, any irregularity in the surface is removed with abrasive discs or a scalpel blade.

Removing the splint

The healing events are monitored radiographically 2-3 weeks after injury. If there is no sign of infection in the bone at the level of the fracture, the splint may be removed.

One year after injury

The tooth reacts normally to sensibility testing and the radiograph shows increasing radio-opacity of the fracture line.

70

Fig. 4.7. **Treatment of a severely extruded root fracture**

This 20-year-old woman has suffered a frontal blow to the left central incisor, resulting in extreme displacement of the coronal fragment.

Examining the displaced coronal fragment

After cleansing of the exposed root surface with saline, it can be seen that the coronal fragment has been forced past the cervical margin of the labial bone plate. The stretched pulp is seen within the socket area.

Repositioning

After a regional block anesthesia, the coronal fragment is repositioned. To guide the root fragment into place, an amalgam carver is inserted beneath the cervical bone margin and used like a shoe horn.

Splinting

The acid-etch technique is employed once optimal repositioning has been verified radiographically. The labial surfaces are etched and a splinting material eg a temporary crown and bridge material is applied. The patient is given penicillin (2 million IU daily for 4 days) to safeguard healing.

71

Diagnosing healing complications

Negative pulpal sensibility, increased separation between fragments as seen radiographically after 3 weeks, together with periradicular radiolucencies (arrows) indicate pulp necrosis in the coronal fragment.

Endodontic treatment of the coronal fragment

A rubber dam is placed over the splinted teeth by punching three overlapping holes. In that way, the splinted teeth can be isolated. The rubber dam can be held in place by wedging a small piece of rubber dam material between the last tooth in the splint and the next unsplinted tooth.

Entering the pulp chamber

After disinfecting the palatal surface of the tooth with a bactericidal solution (e.g. a combination of hydrogen peroxide and chlorhexidine-cetrimonium), an access cavity is prepared and the pulp extirpated. This procedure is not associated with pain and therefore does not require the use of local anesthetic (see also page 122).

Extirpation of the coronal pulp

A barbed broach is inserted into the coronal aspect of the root canal, short of the fracture line, and the pulp extirpated.

CHAPTER 4

Preparation of the root canal

The root canal is rinsed with 1% sodium hypochlorite. A large file is inserted in the root canal as a guide to the level of amputation. A slight pain response will be elicited from the patient when vital tissue at the fracture level is reached. This level should NEVER be exceeded during mechanical preparation.

Obturating the root canal

To induce hard tissue closure of the coronal aspect of the "fracture foramen," calcium hydroxide paste (e.g. Calasept®, Scandia Dental) is used initially as a root canal dressing. The paste is carried into the root canal with a lentulo spiral and condensed with paper points.

Sealing the root canal

A small cotton pellet is placed in the coronal aspect of the canal, approximately 2 mm from the oral surface of the access cavity. The margins of the access cavity are cleansed of calcium hydroxide paste. Thereafter, the cavity is sealed with fortified zinc oxide eugenol cement or glass ionomer cement. A radiograph is taken upon completion of treatment. It should be noted that calcium hydroxide paste has the same radioopacity as dentin.

Follow-up

After 2 weeks, the calcium hydroxide interim dressing is replaced with the final root filling. MTA® can be used to provide an 'apical' stop at the fracture level prior to gutta percha. It should be noted that a setting time of 4-6 hours is necessary prior to condensing gutta percha against the MTA® stop. The clinical and radiographic situation is shown 1 year after injury where the tooth has been restored with a composite resin build-up and the root canal filled with gutta percha.

ROOT FRACTURE

Essentials

- Take radiographs with various angulations to diagnose fracture type and location.
- Reposition the coronal fragment and use splinting for 3 weeks.
- Check for pulpal complications after 3 weeks, 6 weeks and 3 months.
- If pulp necrosis occurs, as indicated radiographically by resorption of bone at the level of the fracture, extirpate the pulp to the level of the fracture and use calcium hydroxide as an interim dressing for 2 weeks. A definitive gutta percha filling can then be made using MTA® as the 'apical' stop at fracture level.

Prognosis

Pulp necrosis is infrequent (approximately 25%) and is related to displacement of the coronal fragment and mature root formation. Progressive root resorption (i.e. inflammatory resorption, ankylosis) is rare. However, resorption within the root canal, is a stage of fracture healing is a frequent finding (60%); but requires no treatment.

74

Fig. 4.8. **Pulp survival after root fracture in teeth with open apices according to type of luxation injury** (after Andreasen et al. 1989).

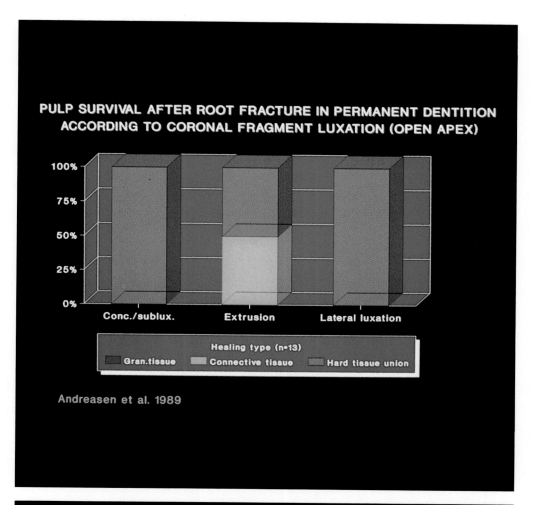

Fig. 4.9. **Pulp survival after root fracture in teeth with closed apices according to type of luxation injury** (after Andreasen et al. 1989).

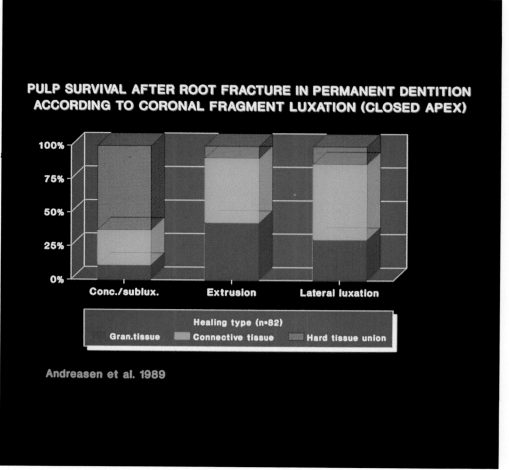

ROOT FRACTURE

CHAPTER 5

Concussion and subluxation

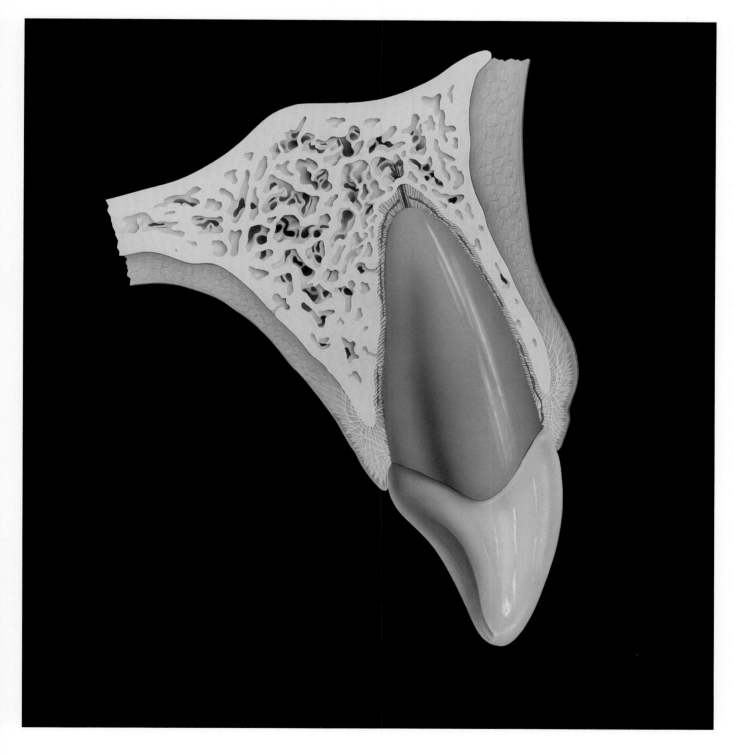

CONCUSSION AND SUBLUXATION

Fig. 5.1. **Mechanism of concussion injury**
A frontal impact leads to hemorrhage and edema in the periodontal ligament.

Fig. 5.2. **Mechanism of sub-luxation injury**
If the impact has greater force, periodontal ligament fibers may be torn, resulting in loosening of the injured tooth.

CONCUSSION AND SUBLUXATION

Pattern of injury and diagnosis

These injuries represent minor injuries to the periodontal ligament and pulp caused by an acute impact (Fig. 5.1). In case of *concussion*, the impact can result in hemorrhage and edema within the periodontal ligament, rendering the tooth tender to percussion and mastication. However, as periodontal ligament fibers are intact, the tooth is firm in its socket and there is no bleeding from the gingival sulcus. Radiographically, there is no sign of pathology (Fig. 5.3). The neurovascular supply to the pulp is usually unaffected by the trauma, usually responding normally to electrometric sensibility testing at the time of injury (see also Appendix 3, page 178).

Greater impact to the tooth will result in *subluxation*, whereby some periodontal ligament fibers will be ruptured and the tooth loosened, but not displaced (Fig. 5.2). There is often slight bleeding from the gingival sulcus (Fig. 5.3).

Treatment

The treatment of both types of injury consists of relief of occlusal interferences (Fig. 5.4) and ordination of a soft diet for approximately 2 weeks. Splinting of the involved teeth is not necessary, but might be desired for the comfort of the patient. If performed,

Fig. 5.3. **Clinical and radiographic features of concussion and subluxation**
The right and left maxillary central incisors have received a blow and are tender to percussion. The right central incisor is firm in its socket (concussion). While the left central incisor is loose with bleeding from the gingival sulcus (subluxation).

80

the teeth should be immobilized for not more than 2 weeks. However, fixation does not appear to promote healing. In the case of multiple tooth injuries, the splinting period will be dictated by the needs of the more severe injuries.

Follow-up procedure

Due to the slight risk of pulp necrosis, sensibility testing should be performed at the time of injury and 1 and 2 months after trauma.

General prognosis

Due to an associated injury to the blood vessels at the root apex, pulp necrosis may occur especially in teeth with a narrow apical foramen (Figs. 5.5 and 5.7). Root resorption, however, is very rare (Figs. 5.6. and 5.8).

Fig. 5.4. **Treatment of injury**
Relief of occlusal interference by selective grinding of opposing teeth is a treatment alternative.

CONCUSSION AND SUBLUXATION

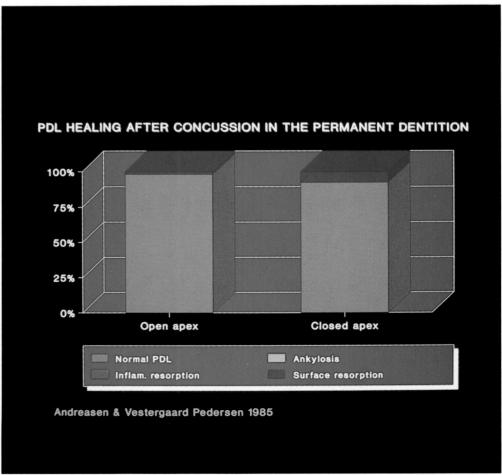

82

Fig. 5.7. **Pulp survival after subluxation** (after Andreasen & Vestergaard Pedersen 1985).

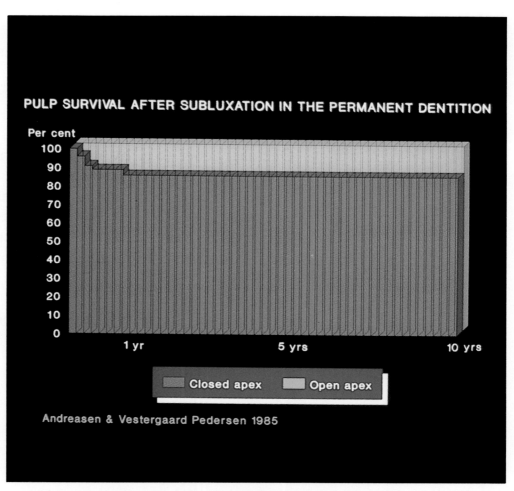

Fig. 5.8. **Periodontal healing after subluxation** (after Andreasen & Vestergaard Pedersen 1985).

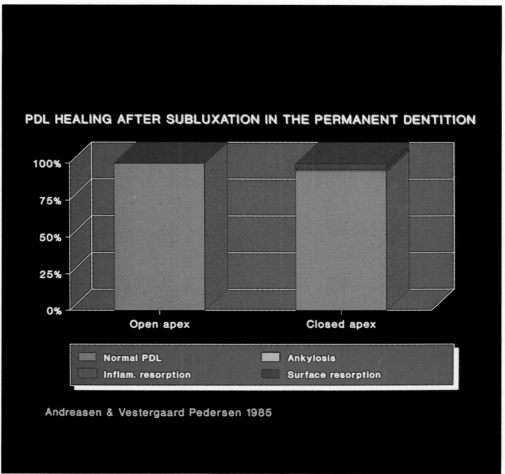

CONCUSSION AND SUBLUXATION

Essentials

- A *concussed* tooth is tender to percussion due to edema and hemorrhage in the PDL.
- A *subluxated* tooth is tender to percussion and also abnormally loose, due to rupture of PDL fibers.

Treatment consists of:

- Occlusal relief (e.g. by selective grinding of opposing teeth) and a soft diet.
- Immobilization of the injured teeth may be appropriate for patient comfort. However, splinting does not appear to promote healing. The fixation period is 2 weeks, unless otherwise dictated by more severe injuries in the dental arch.

Prognosis

There is only a minimal risk of pulp necrosis and even less risk of progressive root resorption.

Extrusion and lateral luxation

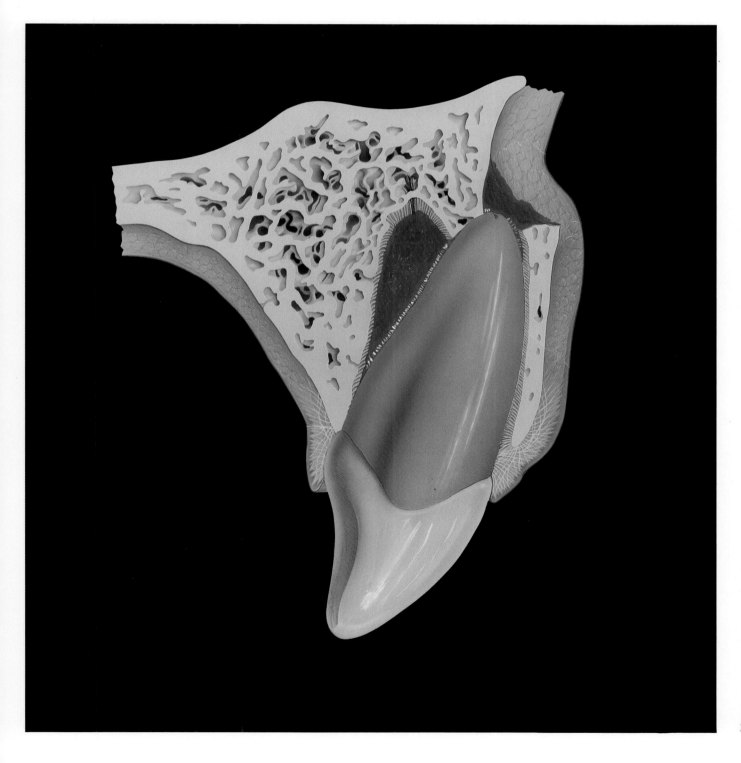

Fig. 6.1. **Pathogenesis of extrusive luxation**
Oblique forces displace the tooth out of its socket. Only the gingival fibers palatally prevent the tooth from being avulsed. Both the PDL and the neurovascular supply to the pulp are severed.

86

Fig. 6.2. **Pathogenesis of lateral luxation**

Horizontal forces displace the crown palatally and the apex labially. Apart from severance of the PDL and the neurovascular supply to the pulp, compression of the PDL is found on the palatal aspect of the root.

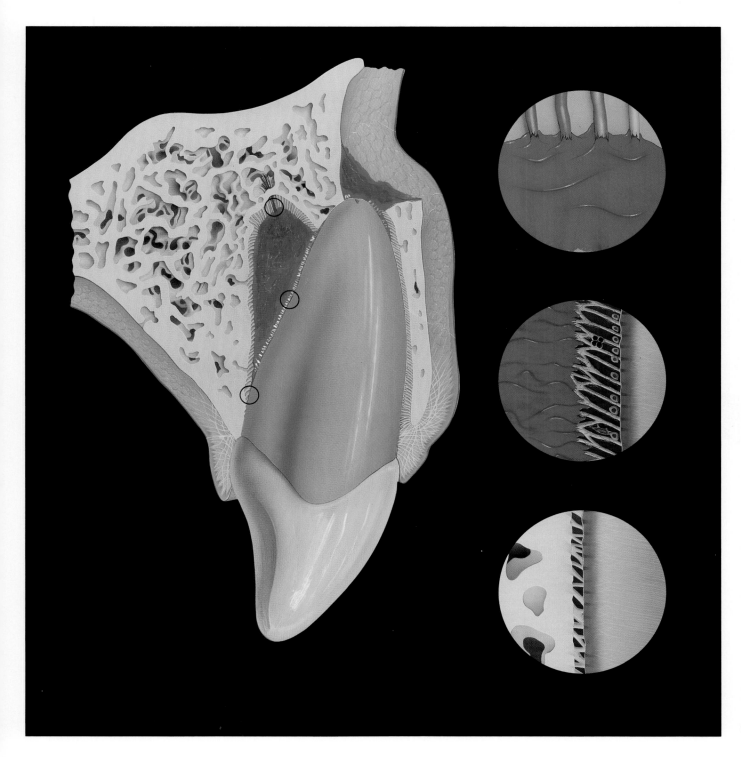

Fig. 6.3. **Clinical and radiographic features of extrusive luxation**
The occlusal (OI) or bisecting angle (BI) radiographic technique is almost equally useful in revealing displacement. PH and PA indicates the appearance after horizontal and axial photographic demonstration.

Fig. 6.4. **Clinical and radiographic features of lateral luxation**
The occlusal radiographic exposure and the eccentric bisecting angle exposure are more useful than an orthoradial bisecting angle exposure in revealing displacement.

Pattern of injury and diagnosis

In these two types of injury, there is a combined periodontal and pulpal injury. In the case of *extrusion*, the acute impact forces the tooth out of its socket, while the palatal periodontal ligament fibers prevent total avulsion (Fig. 6.1). In *lateral luxation*, a horizontal impact forces the crown palatally and the apex labially. Both movements result in contusion or fracture of the alveolar socket walls. Lateral luxation thus creates a complex of compression and rupture zones in the periodontal ligament, pulp and bone (Fig. 6.2).

Clinically, the *extruded* tooth is displaced axially out of its socket and is extremely loose, being held in place by a few intact

Fig. 6.5. **Treatment principles of extrusive luxation: repositioning and splinting**

gingival fibers palatally. Radiographically, a periapical bisecting angle exposure is as useful as an occlusal exposure (Fig. 6.3).

Clinically, the crown of the *laterally luxated tooth* is usually displaced horizontally, with the tooth locked firmly in the new position, thereby eliciting a high metallic percussion (ankylosis) tone (see also Appendix 3, page 178). Radiographic demonstration is entirely dependent upon angulation of the central beam. Thus, a standard orthoradial periapical bisecting angle technique will usually fail to disclose displacement, due to overlapping of the root of the tooth and bone; whereas a more occlusally or eccentrically oriented exposure will tend to come between the root of the tooth and the empty socket, thus revealing the true nature of the injury (Fig. 6.4).

Healing subsequent to *extrusion* depends upon whether repositioning has been optimal. If so, pulpal revascularization and healing will take place as described for replantation. If repositioning has been less than optimal, revascularization will be retarded both in the pulp and periodontal ligament. In a tooth with immature root formation, arrested root development can be expected due to irreversible damage to the Hertwig's epithelial root sheath.

Healing after *lateral luxation* is entirely dependent upon the complex healing pattern resulting from the combined pulpal and periodontal injuries. Thus, the final outcome can range from pulpal and periodontal regeneration/repair to infected pulp necrosis and external root resorption and loss of gingival attachment. The exact circumstances leading to these complications have not yet been identified.

Treatment

Treatment consists of atraumatic repositioning and fixation which prevents excessive movement during the healing period. The value of antibiotic therapy is thus far unknown.

Repositioning of *extruded* incisors is achieved by a slow and steady apical pressure which gradually displaces the coagulum formed between the root apex and floor of the socket as the tooth is moved apically. Thereafter, an acid-etch splint is applied and maintained for 2-3 weeks (Figs. 6.5 and 6.6).

Laterally luxated incisors should be repositioned with as little force as possible (Figs. 6.7 and 6.8). Thus, careful planning is decisive for the repositioning sequence. The general principles follow that of repositioning of tooth segments after fracture of the alveolar process; that is, freeing the apical lock in the cortical labial bone plate (see Chapter 9). This can be achieved either by digital pressure or by the use of forceps, whereafter the tooth is repositioned apically. Digital pressure is presumably the gentlest **91**

Fig. 6.6. Diagnosis and treatment of extrusive luxation
This 17-year-old man has extruded the left central incisor and avulsed the lateral incisor, which could not be retrieved.

Mobility and percussion test
The tooth is very mobile and can be moved in horizontal and axial direction. The percussion test reveals slight tenderness and there is a dull percussion tone.

Sensibility testing and radiographic examination
The tooth does not respond to sensibility testing. The radiographic examination shows coronal displacement of the tooth.

Repositioning
The tooth is gently pushed back into its socket. Thereafter the labial surfaces of both central incisors are etched in preparation for splinting.

Applying splinting material
After rinsing the labial surfaces with water and drying with compressed air, the splinting material (Protemp®, Espe Corp.) is applied.

Polishing the splint
The surface of the splint is smoothed with abrasive discs and contact with the gingiva removed with a straight scalpel blade.

The finished splint
Note that the splint allows optimal oral hygiene in the gingival region which is the most likely port of entry for bacteria which may complicate periodontal and pulpal healing.

Suturing the gingival wound
The gingival wound is closed with interrupted silk sutures. The final radiograph shows optimal repositioning of the tooth.

EXTRUSION AND LATERAL LUXATION

treatment. In this context, correct positioning of the clinician is essential in successful repositioning with digital pressure. Thus, if the operator stands slightly behind the patient, it is possible to palpate the displaced apex in the sulcular fold and with steady pressure force it free of its bony lock. Often a click will be heard as the apex is freed. It is then possible to reposition the tooth. An acid-etch splint is then applied for 3 weeks (Fig. 6.8).

With respect to repositioning of *extruded* teeth, it is not necessary to administer an anesthetic as repositioning can be achieved rather easily with minimum discomfort to the patient. However, it is recommended that anesthetics be used prior to repositioning of *laterally luxated* incisors. This can be accomplished by using an infraorbital regional block on the affected side.

At the time of repositioning, the laterally luxated incisor might appear firm in its position and fixation seem unnecessary. However, it should be considered that temporary breakdown of the marginal bone may occur within 2-4 weeks, resulting in looseness of the luxated tooth and thus requiring prolonged splinting (6-8 weeks) for patient comfort (see later).

Fig. 6.7. **Treatment principles for lateral luxation: repositioning and splinting**

CHAPTER 6

Fig. 6.8. **Diagnosis and treatment of lateral luxation**

This 23-year-old man suffered a lateral luxation of the left central incisor.

Percussion test

Percussion of the injured tooth reveals a high metallic sound.

Mobility and sensibility testing

Mobility testing, using either digital pressure or alternating pressure of two instrument handles facially and orally, reveals no mobility of the injured tooth. There is no response to pulpal sensibility testing.

Radiographic examination

A steep occlusal radiographic exposure revealed, as expected, more displacement than the bisecting angle technique. A lateral radiograph reveals the associated fracture of the labial bone plate (arrow).

EXTRUSION AND LATERAL LUXATION

Anesthesia

An infraorbital regional block is placed and supplemented with anesthesia of the nasopalatinal nerve.

Repositioning

The tooth is repositioned initially by forcing the displaced apex past the labial bone lock and thereby disengaging the root. Thereafter, axial pressure apically will bring the tooth back to its original position. It should be remembered that the palatal aspect of the marginal bone has also been displaced at the time of impact. This must be repositioned with digital pressure to ensure optimal periodontal healing.

Verifying repositioning and splinting with the acid-etch technique

Occlusion is checked and a radiograph taken to verify adequate repositioning. The incisal one-third of the labial aspect of the injured and adjacent teeth are acid-etched (30 seconds) with phosphoric acid gel.

Preparing the splinting material

The etchant is removed with a 20 seconds water spray. The labial enamel is dried with compressed air, revealing the mat, etched surface.

96

Applying the splinting material

A temporary crown and bridge material (e.g. Protemp®) is then applied. Surplus material can be removed after polymerization using a straight scalpel blade or abrasive discs.

Three weeks after injury

At this examination, a radiograph is taken to evaluate periodontal and pulpal healing. That is, neither periapical radiolucency nor breakdown of supporting marginal bone, as compared to the radiograph taken after repositioning.

Splint removal

The splint is removed using fissure burs, by reducing the splinting material interproximally and thereafter thinning the splint uniformly across its total span. Once thinned out, the splint can be removed using a sharp explorer.

Six months after injury

After 6 months, there is a slight sensibility reaction and normal radiographic conditions.

EXTRUSION AND LATERAL LUXATION

Follow-up procedures

The splint may be removed 2-3 weeks after *extrusion*. Three weeks after *lateral luxation* and prior to splint removal, a radiograph is taken to ascertain healing. Due to the extent of trauma, osteoclastic activity may result in a temporary breakdown of the marginal bone, seen as a rarefaction of the marginal periodontium (Fig. 6.9). In this case, it may be necessary to maintain fixation for up to 2 months. Optimal oral hygiene is also necessary during this period. If such changes are not present, the splint may be removed after 3 weeks (see also Appendix 4, page 179).

External inflammatory root resorption may also occur, requiring immediate endodontic therapy with calcium hydroxide as an interim dressing (see page 122).

Also at this time, sensibility testing should be performed. An observation period of up to 12 months or more can pass before a positive response to pulp testing can be expected in these teeth.

General prognosis

The prognosis for extruded and laterally luxated teeth with respect to pulpal and periodontal healing depends upon the stage of root development at the time of injury (Figs. 6.10 to 6.13).

Fig. 6.9. **Transient marginal breakdown**
In this case, temporary loss of marginal bone support is seen 3 weeks after injury, which was later followed by reformation of supporting bone.

Day 0   Day 0   3 weeks   6 weeks   1 year   1 year

Fig. 6.10. **Pulpal healing after extrusive luxation** (after Andreasen & Vestergaard Pedersen 1985).

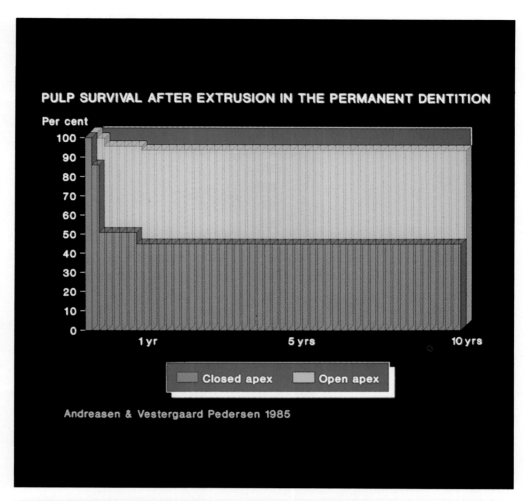

Fig. 6.11. **Periodontal healing after extrusive luxation** (after Andreasen & Vestergaard Pedersen 1985).

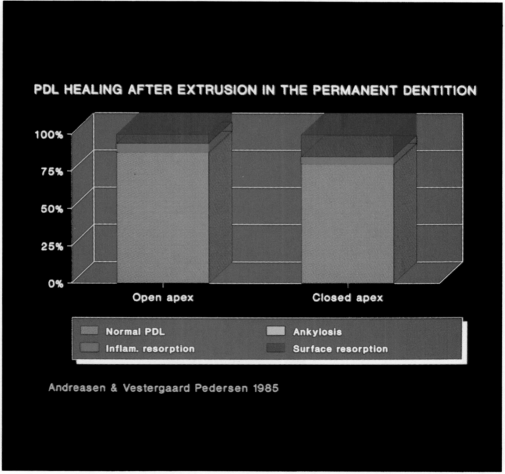

EXTRUSION AND LATERAL LUXATION

Fig. 6.12. **Pulpal healing after lateral luxation** (after Andreasen & Vestergaard Pedersen 1985).

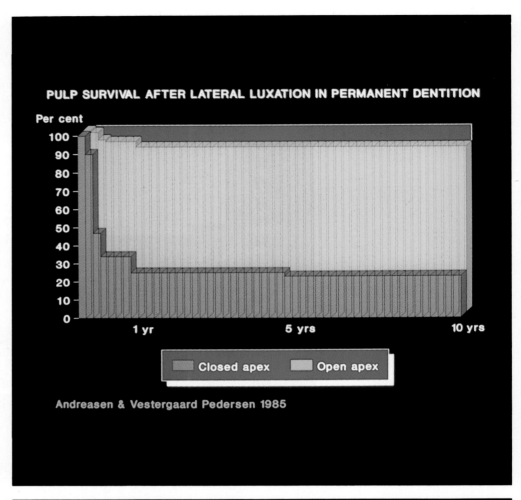

Fig. 6.13. **Periodontal healing after lateral luxation** (after Andreasen & Vestergaard Pedersen 1985).

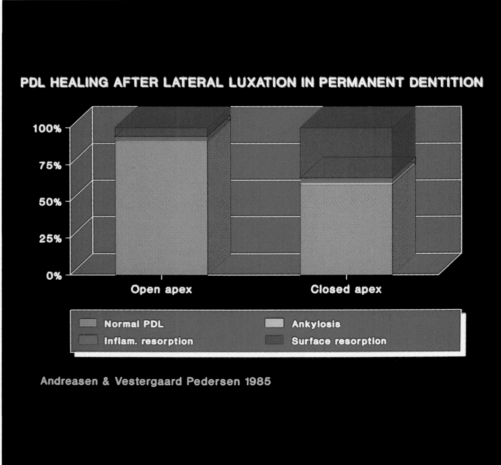

100

Essentials

- **Extrusive luxation** represents a rupture of the PDL and the pulp.
- **Lateral luxation** represents a rupture of the PDL and the pulp as well as injury to the labial and/or palatal alveolar bone plate.
- In both cases, healing includes both PDL repair and usually pulpal revascularization.

Treatment consists of:

- Atraumatic repositioning and fixation.
- In the case of lateral luxation, administration of local anesthetic is necessary prior to repositioning.
- Radiographic examination after 2-3 weeks prior to splint removal.

If radiographic examination reveals no sign of marginal breakdown, the splint can be removed. Otherwise further controls are necessary.

If radiographic examination reveals inflammatory resorption of the bone and root, immediate endodontic therapy is required.

Prognosis

There is considerable risk of pulp necrosis in both luxation categories, especially in teeth with mature root formation. Progressive root resorption is rare after extrusion (Fig. 6.11); but can occur following lateral luxation (Fig. 6.13).

EXTRUSION AND LATERAL LUXATION

Intrusion

103

Fig. 7.1. **Pathogenesis of intrusion**
Axial impact leads to extensive injury to the pulp and periodontium.

Pattern of injury and diagnosis

In this type of injury, maximum damage has occurred to pulp and supporting structures, as the tooth has been driven into the alveolar process due to an axially directed impact (Fig. 7.1). The resulting damage is dependent upon the age of the patient.

In the adult dentition, diagnosis of intrusive luxation is primarily dependent upon the difference in incisal height of the affected and adjacent non-affected teeth (Fig. 7.2). In the mixed dentition, diagnosis is more difficult, as the intrusion can mimic a tooth under eruption. The percussion test, however, will reveal whether the tooth in question is under eruption (a dull tone) or locked into bone (a high metallic tone, pathognomonic for intrusion or lateral luxation, see Appendix 3, page 178) (Fig. 7.3).

Healing after intrusion is usually complicated, as the extensive injury to the PDL can lead to progressive external root resorption (ankylosis). Likewise, damage to the pulp bears with it the risk of inflammatory resorption. Treatment should, therefore, be directed towards eliminating or reducing the extent of both of these healing complications.

Fig. 7.2. **Intrusion of a tooth with completed root formation**
The difference in the level of the incisal edge, as well as the apical shift of the cemento-enamel junction indicates intrusion.

INTRUSION

Fig. 7.3. **Intrusion of a tooth with incomplete root formation**

The semi-erupted position of the tooth leaves doubt about whether the tooth is under eruption or intruded from a more coronal position. A high percussion (ankylosis) tone reveals the intrusion.

Fig. 7.4. **Treatment principles of intrusions: spontaneous eruption or orthodontic extrusion**

Treatment

Treatment principles for intruded permanent incisors are entirely dependent upon the stage of root development (Figs. 7.4 and 7.5). In the case of immature root formation, spontaneous re-eruption can be anticipated. However if eruption has not yet begun after 10 days a local anesthetic can be administered and the tooth luxated slightly with a forceps. During this process, the crushed cervical bone is usually repaired. As spontaneous re-eruption can take up to several months, it is of utmost importance that pulpal healing is constantly monitored (i.e. radiographically).

In cases where a periapical radiolucency or inflammatory root resorption develop, it is essential that the infected pulp be extirpated as soon as the healing complication is diagnosed and the root canal dressed with calcium hydroxide paste. It should be remembered that pulp necrosis is a very frequent finding after intrusion, irrespective of stage of root development.

Due to frequent loss of marginal bone and ankylosis following this procedure, total surgical repositioning at the time of injury is not recommended.

Fig. 7.5. **Spontaneous eruption of two intruded incisors**
Clinical and radiographic condition in a 7-year-old girl after an axial impact.

Initial eruption
Condition 6 weeks later, after onset of eruption.

Follow-up, 1 year after injury
Eruption is complete.

107

Fig. 7.6. Orthodontic extrusion of an intruded incisor
Clinical and radiographic condition in an 22-year-old woman after an axial impact.

Covering exposed dentin
The exposed dentin of both central incisors is covered with a hard-setting calcium hydroxide cement (e.g. Dycal®) and composite.

Applying orthodontic traction
A 0.5 mm thick semi-rigid orthodontic wire is bent to follow the curvature of the dental arch, including two adjacent teeth on either side of the intruded incisor. The orthodontic wire is fastened to the adjacent teeth using an acid-etch technique. In the area where elastic traction is exerted, a coil spring (e.g. 0.228 x 0.901, Elgiloy) is placed in order to prevent slippage of the elastic.

Placing the bracket
A bracket is placed on the labial surface and the fractured incisal edge is covered with a temporary crown and bridge material.

Orthodontic traction

Elastic traction of 70-100 grams is activated. The direction of traction should extrude the tooth out of its socket in a purely axial direction.

Extrusion initiated

After approximately 10 days, osteoclastic activity around the intruded tooth has usually resulted in loosening and extrusion can then occur. If extrusion has not yet begun after 10 days, a local anesthetic is administered and the tooth is luxated slightly with a forceps. After 2-3 weeks, a rubber dam is applied, the pulp extirpated and the root canal is filled with calcium hydroxide paste.

Extrusion complete

After 4 weeks, the intruded tooth is extruded to its original position and the tooth retained in its new position for 2-4 weeks. Thereafter, the orthodontic appliance can be removed.

Crown restoration

The fractured crowns are restored with composite resin.

In the case of completed root development, spontaneous re-eruption is unpredictable and orthodontic extrusion is therefore indicated (Fig. 7.6). Extrusion should be accomplished over a period of 2-3 weeks in order to permit endodontic therapy prior to the radiographic appearance of inflammatory root resorption. As pulp necrosis following intrusion of mature teeth has been found with nearly 100% frequency, prophylactic pulp extirpation is indicated.

Follow-up procedures

Continuous clinical and radiographic monitoring is necessary following this trauma entity as pulpal and periodontal healing complications are so frequent.

Fig. 7.7. **Pulp survival after intrusion** (after Andreasen & Vestergaard Pedersen 1985).

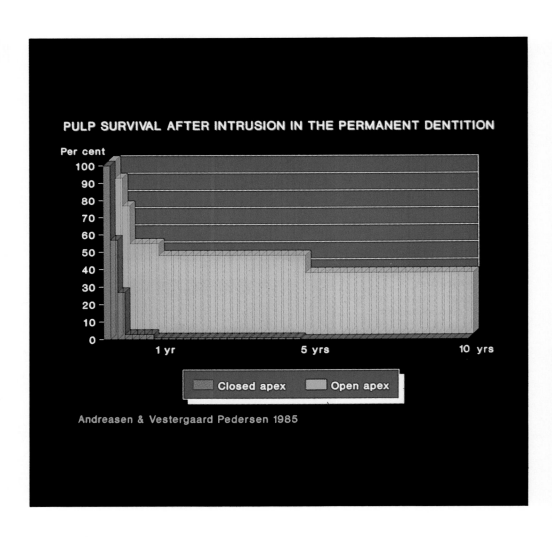

CHAPTER 7

General prognosis

With respect to pulp survival, only teeth with immature root formation have been shown to demonstrate pulp survival following intrusion (Fig. 7.7). With respect to periodontal healing, there is a high risk of root resorption (58% for teeth with immature root formation and 70% for teeth with mature root formation) (Fig. 7.8). Moreover, some teeth have been found to demonstrate ankylosis as late as 5 or 10 years following injury, therefore requiring extended follow-up periods.

Fig. 7.8. **Periodontal healing after intrusion** (after Andreasen & Vestergaard Pedersen 1985).

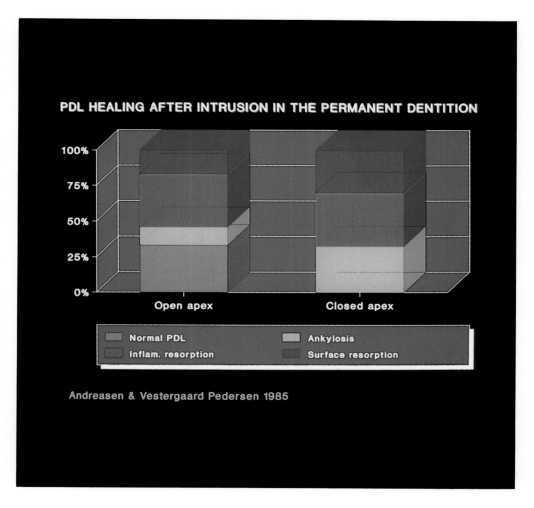

INTRUSION

Essentials

- Intrusion is the result of an axial, apical impact and results in extensive damage to the pulp and PDL.
- Treatment.
- **Immature root formation**

At time or injury, loosen the tooth slightly, with forceps from its bony lock.

Await spontaneous re-eruption, which usually takes 2-4 months.

Monitor pulpal healing radiographically 3, 4 and 6 weeks after injury.
- **Mature root formation**

Await spontaneous re-eruption or extrude orthodontically over a period of 2-3 weeks.

Extirpate the pulp 2 weeks after injury, using calcium hydroxide paste as an interim dressing.

Root fill with a permanent gutta percha filling 2 weeks after use of calcium hydroxide.

Prognosis

There is a high risk of pulp necrosis and progressive root resorption, especially in teeth with mature root formation.

Avulsion injury

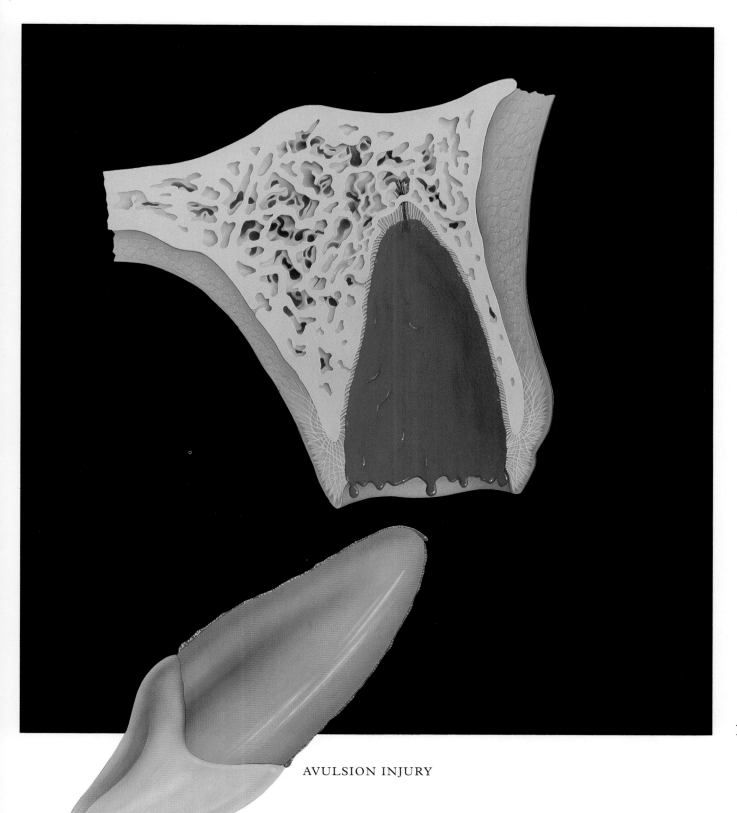

AVULSION INJURY

Fig. 8.1. **Mechanism of avulsion**
Frontal impacts lead to avulsion with subsequent damage to both the pulp and periodontal ligament.

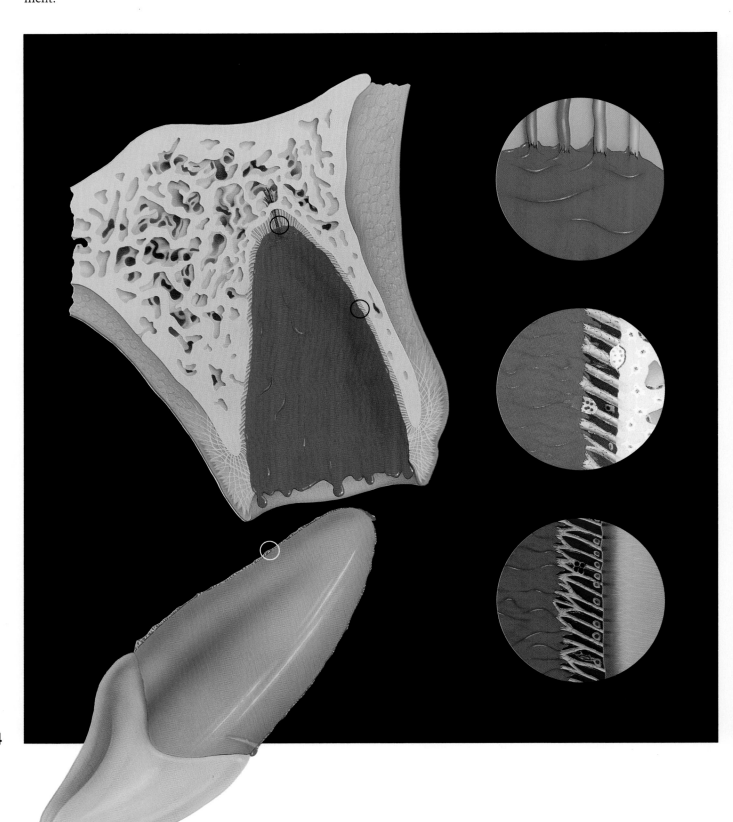

Pattern of injury and diagnosis

Avulsion of permanent teeth is most common in the young dentition, where root development is still incomplete and the periodontium very resilient. Under these circumstances, even slight horizontal impacts may result in total dislocation of the tooth. The outcome of an eventual replantation procedure is almost entirely dependent upon the extraalveolar period and extraalveolar handling. Emphasis will, therefore, be placed on describing treatment methods which optimize healing of the periodontal ligament as well as the pulp.

The basic requirements for optimal healing are that the tooth is out of its socket for as short a period as possible, that the extraalveolar storage is in a physiologic medium and that contamination of the tooth is eliminated, reduced or controlled by antibiotics. If these conditions are met, the following healing events can be expected: Healing is accomplished by revascularization of the severed periodontal ligament, splicing of the ruptured Sharpey's fibers, formation of a new gingival attachment and, finally, revascularization and reinnervation of the pulp.

The *gingival attachment* is re-established 1 week after injury, including splicing of the ruptured gingival fibers (Fig. 8.2). Intraalveolar *periodontal ligament* revascularization is also complete and splicing of PDL fibers initiated 1 week after injury. After 2 weeks, periodontal ligament repair is so advanced that the perio-

Fig. 8.2. **Healing events 2 weeks after replantation**
Most of the intraalveolar periodontal fibers have healed. Pulpal revascularization has reached mid-root level.

115

dontium has regained about two-thirds of its original strength (Fig. 8.2).

Pulpal revascularization begins 4 days after injury and proceeds at a rate of approximately 0.5 mm per day. This would imply that an entire incisor pulp in a young individual can be revascularized within 30-40 days.

In case of physical damage or bacterial contamination to the pulp or periodontal ligament, aberrations in healing will occur. Thus if there is minor damage to the innermost layer of the periodontal ligament, this site will be resorbed by macrophages and osteoclasts, resulting in a superficial excavation of the root surface

Fig. 8.3. **Healing with minor injury to the periodontal ligament resulting in repair related resorption (surface resorption)**
The injury site is resorbed by macrophages and osteoclasts. Subsequent repair takes place with formation of new cementum and Sharpey's fibers.

CHAPTER 8

(Fig. 8.3). After some weeks, this resorption cavity will be repaired by new cementum and Sharpey's fibers. This resorption entity has been termed *repair related resorption* (surface resorption).

In the event that the initial resorption cavity has penetrated cementum and reached the dentinal tubules, toxins from an eventual infection in the root canal or dentinal tubules can be transmitted via the exposed tubules to the root surface (Fig. 8.4). This event will lead to a continuation of the osteoclastic process and progressive resorption of the root surface, ultimately perforating to the root canal. This resorption entity has been termed *infection related resorption* (inflammatory resorption).

Fig. 8.4. **Healing with moderate injury to the periodontal ligament and associated infection in the pulp and/or dentinal tubules resulting in infection related resorption (inflammatory resorption)** The initial injury to the root surface triggers a macrophage and osteoclast attack on the root surface. If the resorption cavity exposes infected tubules which can transmit bacterial toxins, the resorptive process is accelerated and granulation tissue ultimately invades the root canal.

On the other hand, if infection in the root canal and the dentinal tubules is eliminated by endodontic therapy, osteoclastic activity is arrested and healing with new cementum and Sharpey's fibers will take place.

In case of moderate to extensive damage to the innermost layer of the periodontal ligament, competitive healing processes will occur, whereby cells from the adjacent intact periodontal ligament will attempt to invade and heal the injury site; just as cells from the opposing alveolar bone will also attempt to fill out the traumatized region with new bone (Fig. 8.5). After approximately 2 weeks, bony invasion creates an ankylosis. This ankylosis will

Fig. 8.5. **Healing after extensive injury to the periodontal ligament resulting in ankylosis related resorption (replacement resorption)**
Ankylosis is formed because healing occurs almost exclusively by cells from the alveolar wall.

CHAPTER 8

due to the inherent remodeling capacity of bone lead to a resorption entity named ankylosis related resorption (replacement resorption), the fate of which depends upon the extent of damage to the periodontal ligament and whether there is any functional movement of the injured tooth during the healing period. If there is only minimal injury to the periodontal ligament and the tooth has not been splinted, function will stimulate osteoclastic removal of the bony bridge (i.e. transient ankylosis).

In the event of more extensive damage, and thereby a larger ankylosis site, functional stimulation will not be able to remove the ankylosis. In this case, ankylosis will be permanent (Fig. 8.5). A gradual, progressive resorption of the tooth can be expected due to the inherent remodelling of bone. This process is very active in children, whereby survival of the injured tooth can be limited to only a few years; whereas, in adults, replacement resorption is significantly slower, allowing the affected tooth to survive 10 – and sometimes even 20 – years or more.

If, during pulpal revascularization, bacteria gain access to the the ischemic pulp tissue, either via a gap in the periodontal ligament, the blood stream (anachoresis) or dentinal tubules as after crown fracture, the revascularization process will stop and a zone of inflammation, demarcated by leucocytes, will be established. This leucocyte zone will separate the infected, ischemic pulp from the invading healing tissue. If there has also been a concomitant injury to the periodontal ligament, progressive external inflammatory root resorption will result.

Treatment

Following avulsion of permanent incisors there are basically 3 treatment alternatives: immediate replantation, delayed replantation or no replantation. Each alternative is based on length of time and conditions of extraalveolar storage and age of the patient.

Immediate replantation, in all patient groups, where extraalveolar period is under 60 minutes and storage media physiological (e.g. physiological saline, saliva, milk).
Delayed replantation, with accompanying extraoral fluoride treatment (see later), in patients with completed root development (closed apices) and a **dry** extraalveolar period greater than 60 min.
No replantation, in patients with open apices and a **dry** extraalveolar period greater than 60 min., as well as patients with severe periodontal conditions and gross, untreated carious lesions of the involved teeth.
However, if the avulsed tooth has been soon after trauma placed in a physiological storage medium, the time scale for successful **119**

replantation can be considerably extended. Thus, the following storage media have been shown to permit both periodontal and pulpal healing: physiologic saline, tissue culture media, milk and saliva. A feature common to all of these media is their relative osmotic balance with pulp and periodontal tissues. Avulsed teeth can thus be maintained for hours and in certain media (e.g. modified tissue culture media such as Viaspan® and Dentosafe®) even days before damage to these tissues occurs.

In the case of saliva, however, the extraalveolar period should be limited to a maximum of 2 hours due to the slight hypotonic nature of the media. Moreover, bacteria present in saliva can also have a detrimental effect on later healing.

Cleansing procedures of the root surface also influence healing. Thus, thorough rinsing of the root surface including around the apical foramen with saline should precede replantation in order to remove foreign bodies and bacteria which will stimulate an inflammatory response.

To optimize healing, the alveolus should also be flushed with saline to remove the coagulum. Recent investigations suggest that the presence of a coagulum in the socket at the time of replantation can enhance ankylosis.

Once the root surface and alveolus have been flushed with saline, the tooth can be replanted. This is accomplished using a minimum of pressure, being careful not to further damage the periodontal ligament and pulp. If any resistance is met, the tooth should be placed in saline and the socket visually inspected for possible fractures. Fracture of the socket wall is the most common source of difficulty in replanting avulsed teeth. The fractured bone can usually be repositioned by inserting a flat instrument (e.g. a straight elevator) and remodelling the alveolus. Replantation can then be completed. After repositioning of the tooth, a slightly flexible splint should be applied, such as an acid-etch retained splint of temporary crown and bridge material (e.g. Protemp®, Espe Co.). The splint should be removed after 7 days to allow some functional movement of the replant in order to reduce or eliminate the risk of ankylosis.

Antibiotic and antitetanus therapy

Antibiotic coverage should be given (e.g. pencillin 1000 mg immediately, thereafter 500 mg four times daily for 4 days). Tetanus prophylaxis is assessed according to the immunization status of the patient.

In teeth with complete root formation (i.e. the diameter of the apical foramen is less than 1.0 mm), the pulp should be extirpated and the root canal dressed with pure calcium hydroxide (e.g. Calasept®, Scandia Dental) immediately prior to splint

Fig. 8.6. **Replantation of a tooth with completed root formation**

Replantation of an avulsed maxillary right central incisor in a 19-year-old man. Radiographic examination shows no sign of fracture or contusion of the alveolar socket. The tooth was retrieved immediately after injury and kept moist in the oral cavity. Upon admission to the emergency service, the avulsed incisor was placed in physiologic saline.

Rinsing the tooth

The tooth is examined for fractures, position of the level of periodontal attachment and signs of contamination. The tooth is then rinsed with a stream of saline until all visible signs of contamination have been removed. If this is not effective, dirt is carefully removed using a gauze sponge soaked in saline. The coagulum in the alveolar socket is flushed out using a stream of saline.

Replanting the tooth

The tooth is grasped by the crown with forceps and partially replanted in its socket. Replantation is completed using gentle finger pressure. If any resistance is met, the tooth should be removed, placed again in saline and the socket inspected. A straight elevator is then inserted in the socket and an index finger is placed labially. Using lateral pressure, counterbalanced by the finger pressure, the socket wall is repositioned. Replantation can then atraumatically proceed as described.

Splinting

An acid-etch retained splint is applied using the technique described on p. 91. As soon after injury as possible, antibiotic therapy should be instituted. Suggested dosage penicillin 1 million IU immediately, thereafter 2-4 million IU daily for 4 days.

Good oral hygiene is absolutely necessary in the healing period. This includes brushing with a soft tooth brush and chlorhexidine mouth rinse.

Follow-up: endodontic treatment

One week after replantation, the pulp is extirpated prophylactically to avoid external root resorption. A rubber dam is applied by punching 3 overlapping holes in the dam. The dam is held in place by wedging an extra piece of rubber or dental floss between the last splinted tooth and the adjacent non-splinted tooth in the arch.

Extirpating the pulp

After disinfecting the crown of the replanted tooth, an access cavity is prepared to the root canal, its direction following the long axis of the root to allow sufficient mechanical preparation of the entire canal.

The pulp is extirpated by introducing a barbed broach into the midportion of the root canal. A leucocyte zone formed 1-2 mm from the apical foramen will determine the correct amputation level.

Amputation level

The coronal pulp chamber is cleansed of pulpal remnants using a small excavator. Careful instruction to the patient as to when he or she just feels the instrument, will dictate the level of chemomechanical root canal preparation and avoid overinstrumentation and post-operative discomfort. This procedure is not associated with pain and therefore does not require the use of local anesthetic.

Preparing the canal

The root canal is prepared with reamers and files using standard endodontic procedures. During this procedure, the root canal is cleansed using sodium hypochlorite as an irrigating medium.

Placing the calcium hydroxide dressing

After preparation of the root canal, it is flushed with saline. Filling of the root canal with calcium hydroxide paste is facilitated if done in a wet canal. This allows placement of the paste up to the root apex without entrapment of air which could interfere with complete canal obturation. Commercially prepared paste (e.g. Calasept®, Scandia Dental) is injected into the canal and distributed with a lentulo spiral.

Condensing the calcium hydroxide dressing

The paste is condensed slightly with paper points. Filling and condensing is repeated 3 times, whereafter a small cotton pellet is placed into the pulp chamber and compressed apically.

Closing the access cavity

After removing calcium hydroxide residue from the cavity margins with a water spray, the cavity is air-dried and closed (e.g. IRM®, Cavit®, or glass ionomer cement) to prevent microleakage. Radiographically, calcium hydroxide dressing has the same radiodensity as dentin. The dressing is replaced 2 weeks later with a gutta percha root filling. MTA® can be used to achieve an apical stop. However, a setting period of 4-6 hours is necessary prior to condensing gutta percha.

Splint removal

Once the initial endodontic therapy has been completed, the splinting material can be removed using a fissure bur. The splint is thinned out along its entire span, avoiding gross reduction at any single tooth. The remaining shell of resin interproximally can be removed with a scaler while supporting the replanted tooth incisally. The facial enamel surfaces can be polished with pumice at a later date.

AVULSION INJURY

Fig. 8 7. Replanting a tooth with incomplete root formation

This 8-year-old boy has avulsed his maxillary left central incisor. The extraalveolar period was 80 min (5 min dry storage; 45 min in saliva; 30 min in physiologic saline). Due to the very patent apical foramen, revascularization of the pulp is considered possible.

Rinsing the root surface

The tooth is rinsed carefully with a stream of saline from a syringe. Special care is taken to rinse the apical part of the pulp as well.

Replanting the tooth

After cleansing the socket with physiologic saline, the tooth is replanted using the procedure described in the previous case.

Monitoring healing

Clinical findings and the radiographic control of healing performed 3 weeks after replantation reveal an infected pulp necrosis.

Fig. 8.8. **Replanting a tooth with an avital periodontal ligament**

In this 21-year-old man, the tooth has been kept dry for 24 hours. Total and irreversible damage to the PDL and pulp can be expected. Furthermore, there is severe contusion of the alveolar socket. In this situation, delayed replantation (to allow healing of the socket), treatment of the root surface (to make it resistant to ankylosis) and endodontic therapy (to prevent inflammatory resorption) is the treatment of choice.

Treatment of the root surface

The avulsed tooth was in this case kept dry in a refrigerator until healing of the contused socket has taken place. Prior to sodium fluoride treatment, the root surface is rinsed and scraped clean of the dead PDL and the pulp extirpated. The goal of therapy is to incorporate fluoride ions into the dentin and cementum in order to protract the resorption process.

Fluoride treatment of cementum and dentin

The pulp is extirpated and the root canal enlarged to provide access to the fluoride solution along the entire root canal. The tooth is then placed in a 2.4% solution of sodium fluoride (acidulated to pH = 5.5) for 20 min.

Endodontic treatment

After rinsing in saline, the root canal is obturated with gutta percha and a sealer.

Condition of the socket
After 3 weeks, the socket area and the contused gingiva are healed.

Replanting the tooth
The socket is evacuated with excavators and a surgical bur. The tooth is replanted after cleansing with saline to remove excess fluoride solution.

Splinting
The tooth is splinted for 6 weeks in order to create a solid ankylosis. In these cases, where no periodontal ligament exists, ankylosis is the only possible healing modality.

Follow-up
Radiographic follow-up over a 3-year period shows no progression of the ankylosis process.

126

removal. In teeth whose apical foramen is greater than 1.0 mm, pulpal revascularization is possible. The patient should, therefore, be monitored weekly during the 1st month after injury in order to detect early signs of pulpal infection and inflammatory resorption.

Delayed replantation: sodium fluoride treatment of the root surface

In the case of extended extraalveolar periods in adults, an alternative replantation procedure is possible, whereby the replantation becomes "implantation", in that the root surface is treatment with an fluoride solution to make the root surface partly osteoclast resistant and thereby protract the replacement process of any later ankylosis.

Replantation of avulsed teeth is illustrated in Figs. 8.6 to 8.8 for different trauma situations.

Follow-up procedures

Replanted teeth should be monitored at regular intervals based upon stage of root development and those times where healing complications might be diagnosed (see Appendix 4, page 179). Thus, a radiographic examination 3 weeks after replantation will permit diagnosis of inflammatory resorption and periapical radiolucency, both indications of infected pulp necrosis (Fig. 8.9). If the radiographic findings vaguely suggest these events, further examinations at 1-week intervals should be made (i.e. for the 1st month). Otherwise, follow-up again at 6 weeks, 3 months and 6 months after injury. A high percussion tone and diminished mobility will reveal ankylosis earlier than radiographs. However, by 6 to 8 weeks, ankylosis can sometimes be seen radiographically (Fig. 8.10).

Fig. 8.9. Development of inflammatory root resorption and pulp necrosis
Development of external inflammatory root resorption and periapical radiolucency subsequent to replantation. Periapical radiolucency is evident 1 week after replantation and inflammatory root resorption can be detected after 3 weeks.

Day 0   1 week   3 weeks   4 weeks   2 months   3 months

Immediate endodontic therapy with pulpal extirpation and calcium hydroxide root canal dressing will arrest inflammatory root resorption.

General prognosis

The general outcome of replantation of avulsed teeth is shown in graphs related to pulpal and periodontal ligament healing (Figs. 8.11 and 8.12). However, it should be noted that there is a great variation in healing as related to the time and length of dry extra-alveolar storage (Figs. 8.13 and 8.14).

Fig. 8.10. Development of ankylosis
After avulsion in a 25-year-old man, ankylosis could be diagnosed 10 weeks after injury by the percussion test; whereas radiographic diagnosis could be made after 4 months (arrow). Note the slow progression of the resorption process.

| 1 week | 2 months | 4 months | 1 year | 2 years | 10 years |

Fig. 8.11. **Pulpal healing after replantation related to stage of root development** (after Andreasen et al., 1995)

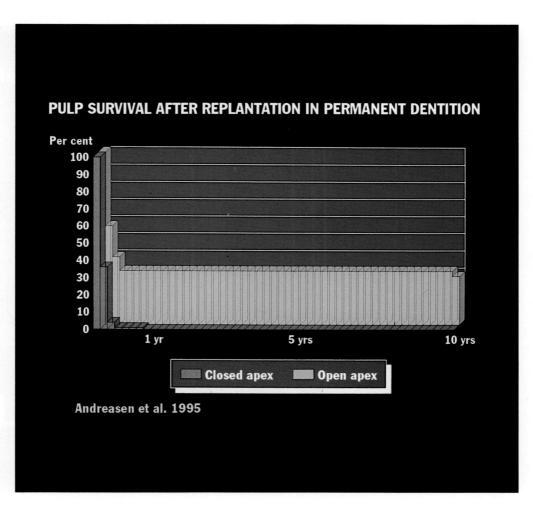

Fig. 8.12. **Periodontal healing after replantation related to stage of root development** (after Andreasen et al., 1995)

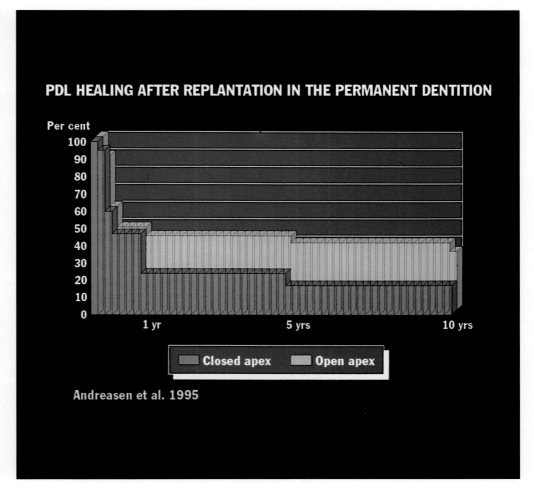

AVULSION INJURY

Fig. 8.13. **Pulpal healing related to dry extraalveolar time** (after Andreasen et al., 1995)

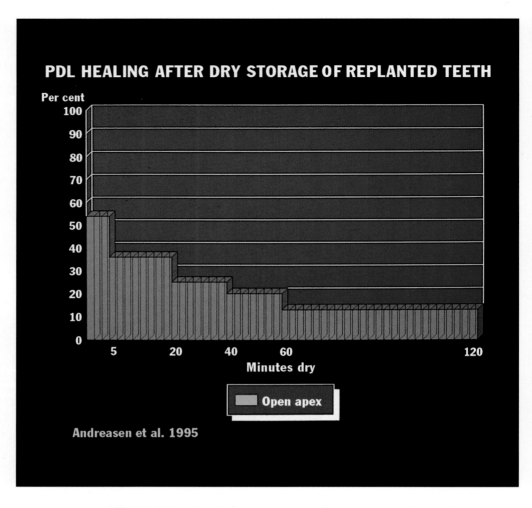

Fig. 8.14. **Periodontal healing related to dry extraalveolar time** (after Andreasen et al., 1995)

CHAPTER 8

Essentials

- Replantation of avulsed teeth can result in successful healing if there has been only minimal damage to the pulp and periodontal ligament.
- The type of extraalveolar storage and length of storage period have an overwhelming effect upon later healing.
- Replantation should be attempted only if the following conditions can be fulfilled:
  - Absence of gross caries and no major loss of periodontal support prior to injury;
  - Physiological storage of the tooth (in the case of an avital PDL, see below).

Replantation procedure

- Place the avulsed tooth in saline;
- Examine the socket area;
- Rinse the periodontal ligament and apical foramen with saline;
- Flush the socket with saline;
- Replant the tooth with gentle finger pressure;
- Splint the tooth for 1 week with a semi-rigid splint;
- Begin antibiotic therapy as soon as possible after injury (e.g. penicillin, 1000 mg, thereafter 500 mg four times daily for 4 days);
- If the patient is not covered for tetanus, tetanus vaccine should be administered.
- In case of incomplete root formation (i.e. diameter of the apical foramen exceeding 1 mm), pulpal revascularization is a possibility.
- In the case of complete root formation, extirpate the pulp at the same appointment as splint removal (i.e. just prior to removal of the splint) and dress the root canal with calcium hydroxide.

- In case of an *avital PDL* (e.g. extraalveolar dry period longer than 1 hour; *only* for patients past active growth), resorption-preventing treatment is indicated:
- Remove the PDL and pulp;
- Place the tooth in 2.4% sodium fluoride solution (acidulated to pH = 5.5) for 20 min.;
- Obturate the root canal with gutta percha and a sealer;
- Replant the tooth;
- Splint for 6 weeks.

Prognosis

Primarily dependent upon extraalveolar period and storage medium. Pulp survival almost nil in teeth with completed root formation and infrequent in teeth with immature root formation. Periodontal ligament healing infrequent and dependent upon the abovementioned factors.

131

Fracture of the alveolar process

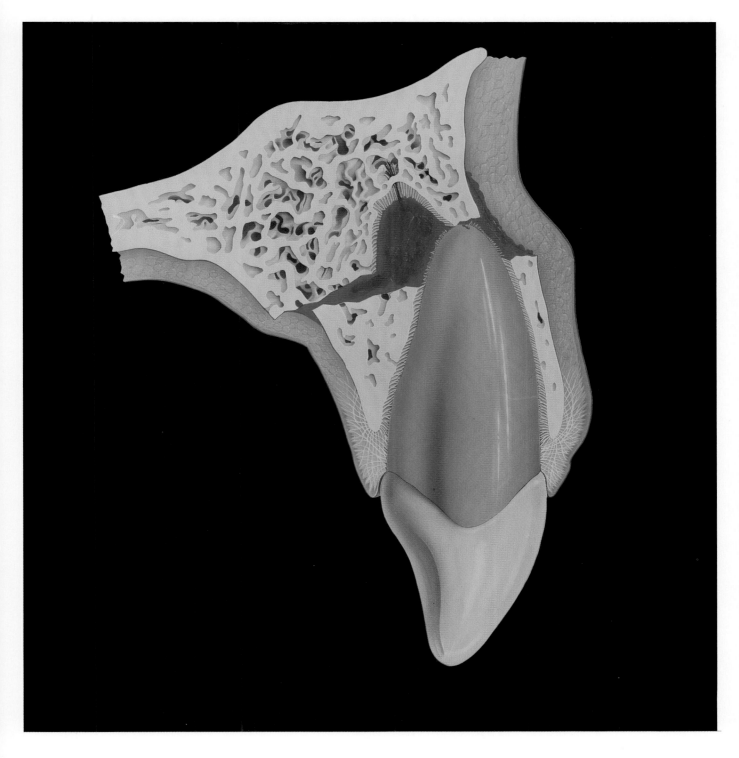

FRACTURE OF THE ALVEOLAR PROCESS

Fig. 9.1. **Fracture of the alveolar process**
Both the PDL and the neurovascular supply to the pulp are severed.

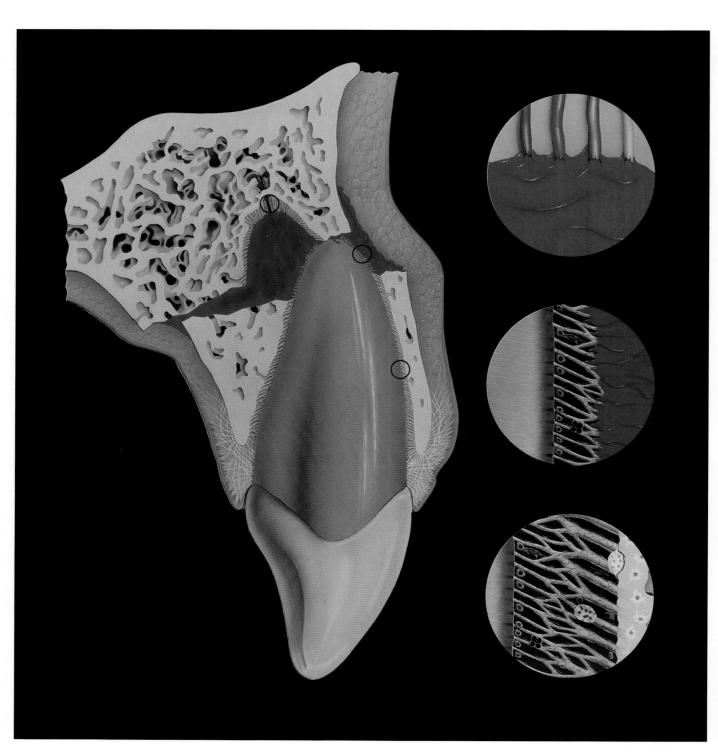

Pattern of injury and diagnosis

Fracture of the alveolar process is in this context limited to a fracture encompassing the entire alveolar process (Fig. 9.1). Partial alveolar fracture, such as fracture of the labial or lingual bone plate are typical sequelae to lateral luxation and therefore described in that chapter.

Alveolar fracture is a result of a heavy impact to the anterior region. Because of the delicate bone structure of the mandibular incisor region, alveolar fractures are often seen in this region. The fracture usually involves 2 or more teeth and generally follows the PDL of an involved tooth in its vertical course. The horizontal component of the fracture can be seen either at the base of the alveolar process free of the apices, at the level of, or coronal to, the apices.

Radiographic demonstration of the entire fracture, including the horizontal and vertical components, is often difficult. Differential diagnosis includes possible root fracture. Thus, multiple radiographs using varying vertical angulations will reveal a fracture line that can move up and down along the root surface in case of an alveolar fracture versus a fracture that remains at the same level of the root in the case of a root fracture.

In this regard, the clinical examination is often more precise in revealing the nature and extent of injury. Thus, when the mobility of one tooth is tested, several teeth move. Also, a hematoma in the adjacent attached gingiva or mucosa is often an indication of alveolar fracture.

Treatment

Treatment principles for fractures of the alveolar process are identical to those for bone fractures in general and consist of repositioning and splinting for 3-4 weeks. With respect to repositioning, the problems involved here are similar to those seen following lateral luxation. That is, the root apices are often locked into the facial aspect of the labial bone plate and thus must be

Fig. 9.2. **Treatment principles of an alveolar fracture: repositioning and splinting**

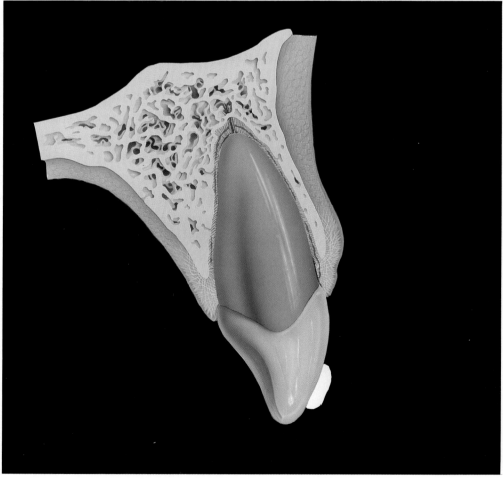

CHAPTER 9

Fig. 9.3. Fracture of the maxillary alveolar process
This 21-year-old woman suffered a fracture of the maxillary alveolar process including the lateral and central incisors.

Anesthetizing the traumatized region
An infraorbital block and infiltration to the incisive canal are necessary prior to repositioning.

Repositioning
With hard finger pressure to the apical region the apices are disengaged. If this is not sufficient then the fragment has to be moved with forceps in a coronal and palatal direction.

Splinting
During curing of the temporary crown and bridge material the patient occludes in order to ensure correct position of the fragment.

FRACTURE OF THE ALVEOLAR PROCESS

further displaced incisally before the tooth and bone segment can be repositioned (Fig. 9.2).

The critical feature in healing of alveolar fractures is pulp related trauma. When the fracture level is apical to the root tips, the vascular supply to the pulp is relatively safe and pulp necrosis rare. In contrast, if the root apices are directly involved in the line of fracture, pulpal healing is jeopardized.

In Fig. 9.3 and 9.4 two examples of repositioning and splinting of alveolar fractures are presented.

Fig. 9.4. Fracture of the mandibular alveolar process
An alveolar fracture involving 4 incisors following collision with the steering wheel by a 25-year-old man during an automobile accident.

Apical lock of the fragment
Attempts at repositioning prove unsuccessful because the apices are locked over the labial bone plate.

Disengagement of the apices
The alveolar fragment is pressed lingually, thereby freeing the apices. Once the apices have been freed, the fragment can be repositioned and the apices will enter their respective sockets.

138

Fig. 9.5. **Pulpal healing after alveolar fracture** (after Andreasen 1970)

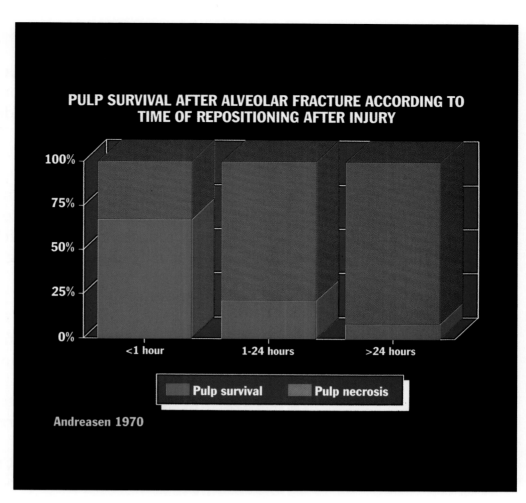

Fig. 9.6. **Periodontal healing after alveolar fracture** (after Andreasen 1970)

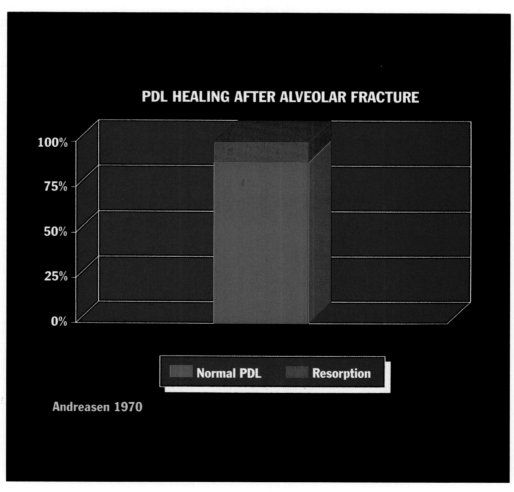

139

FRACTURE OF THE ALVEOLAR PROCESS

Follow-up procedures

The splint can be removed after 3-4 weeks. Due to the frequent occurrence of pulpal and periodontal complications a careful follow-up program is essential (see Appendix 4, page 179).

General prognosis

Very few studies have been performed to ascertain healing after alveolar fractures. To date, the only factor related to pulpal healing has been early repositioning of the fracture (Fig. 9.5). Periodontal healing is usually uneventful (Fig. 9.6).

Essentials

- Verify the extent and position of the fracture clinically and radiographically, using a multiple radiographic exposure technique.
- Use a regional block anesthesia. Determine whether there is an "apical lock", implying that the fragment cannot be completely repositioned.
- In case of an apical lock, the fragment must first be slightly extruded to free the apices. It is then possible to reposition the fragment.
- Splint the fragment for 3-4 weeks, according to the age of the patient.
- Monitor pulpal healing of the involved teeth.

Prognosis

The only predictor for pulp necrosis is late repositioning of the fracture. Root resorption is rare.

Injuries to the primary dentition

INJURIES TO THE PRIMARY DENTITION

Fig. 10.1. **Anatomic relationship between the two dentitions**
The maxilla in a skull of a 3-year-old child. The intimate relation is shown between the primary central incisor and the permanent successor.

Pattern of injury and diagnosis

Injuries to the primary dentition are common. Because of the resilient bone surrounding the primary teeth, injuries usually comprise tooth luxations. The close proximity of the two dentitions represents a risk to the permanent dentition in that energy from the acute impact can easily be transmitted to the developing tooth germ (Figs. 10.1 and 10.2). Moreover, inflammation related to pulpal complications of the displaced tooth may add further injury. In fact, approximately one-half of all primary tooth injuries result in more or less severe disturbances in permanent tooth development. These disturbances range from mineralization disturbances to complete malformation of the tooth germ.

The treatment strategy after injury in the primary dentition is, therefore, dictated by concern for the safety of the permanent dentition. To ensure this, the following treatment demands must be respected.

– To ascertain whether or not the displaced primary incisor has invaded the follicle of the developing permanent tooth germ.

Fig. 10.2. Trauma-related interference with odontogenesis
An intruded primary tooth may be forced into the follicle and disturb the reduced enamel epithelium and secretory ameloblasts, resulting in enamel opacity and/or hypoplasia.

Fig. 10.3. **A parent can assist in stabilizing the child during the radiographic examination**
The parent and child are furnished with lead aprons. One arm is used to hold the child while the other holds the filmholder and stabilizes the child's head against the parent's chest.

Fig. 10.4. **Schematic illustration of the geometric relationship between an intruded primary incisor and the developing tooth germ and the resultant radiographic image. Below, the normal relationship between the primary incisor and developing tooth germ.**

If the primary tooth is intruded AWAY from the developing tooth erm, the radiographic image will be FORESHORTENED. If the primary tooth is intruded INTO the developing tooth germ, the radiographic image will be ELONGATED.

CHAPTER 10

If this has occurred, the primary tooth must be removed.

– To monitor healing in the trauma zone so that secondary damage to the developing permanent tooth can be avoided.

Examination of the traumatized primary dentition consists of a clinical examination as well as a radiographic examination of the traumatized region (see Chapter 1). In the case of small and/or unruly children, adult assistance can be necessary (Fig. 10.3). Radiographic examination is also facilitated if it is possible to adjust kilovoltage on the x-ray unit. Thus, for each 10 kVp increase, exposure time can be reduced by one-half without great sacrifice in quality.

With respect to the first treatment demand, this can only be fulfilled by adequate radiographic technique. Two factors are significant: the radiographic dimension of the intruded incisor and the symmetrical orientation of the permanent tooth germs. Regarding the radiographic dimension of the intruded incisor, it can be seen that an incisor which has invaded the follicle of the permanent tooth germ moves away from the x-ray source and thereby becomes *elongated*. In contrast, a primary incisor which is intruded facially, (i.e. away from the permanent follicle and towards the x-ray source) becomes *foreshortened* (Fig. 10.4).

Fig. 10.5. **Radiographic demonstration of displacement of the developing permanent tooth germ following intrusion of the primary incisor** The distance between the incisal edge and mineralization front of the involved developing tooth germ is shorter than the same distance in the non-involved tooth germ, implying luxation of the involved tooth germ. Although the displaced primary tooth was removed, a slight dilaceration of the permanent crown developed.

INJURIES TO THE PRIMARY DENTITION

Until crown formation is complete and root formation begins, it is possible that intrusion of a primary incisor can lead to displacement of the permanent tooth germ. Unless diagnosed and treated immediately, tooth germ luxation can lead to severe malformation of the crown of the affected permanent tooth. Diagnostic features of tooth germ luxation are the following. If the intruded primary incisor has invaded the follicle of the permanent tooth germ and thereby displaced it, the distance between its incisal edge and the mineralization front will be shorter than the same distance of its counterpart (Fig. 10.5). However, for diagnosis to be valid, the radiograph must be symmetrical with respect to midline alignment. For further illustration of these concepts, see later under treatment of intrusions.

Treatment

Crown fractures
Most fractures consist of chipped enamel or superficial enamel-dentin fractures. In both situations, slight grinding of sharp edges is sufficient. In cases of pulp exposure, a pulpotomy can be performed if the child is cooperative. Otherwise, extraction is the treatment of choice.

Crown-root fractures
In these cases, the pulp is usually involved and extraction is the treatment of choice.

Fig. 10.6. **Root fracture in the primary dentition**
These root fractures occurred at the age of 4 years. Due to severe displacement, both coronal fragments were extracted. The root tips remained in situ and were resorbed normally.

Root fractures

These cases can be treated conservatively. Splinting is usually difficult or impossible to perform in the primary dentition (due to diminutive tooth size and lack of patient cooperation). Healing must, therefore, occur despite mobility at the fracture line, usually resulting in interposition of connective tissue. In some instances, infection will occur in the coronal pulp, in which case it is important to consider that only the coronal fragment need be extracted and that the apical fragment can be left to resorb physiologically (Fig. 10.6).

Extrusive luxation

This injury occurs quite often due to frontal impacts hitting the anterior region. The involved teeth are usually displaced in a combined axial and lingual direction being attached by the palatal or lingual gingiva. The treatment of choice is repositioning supplemented with splinting if the child is cooperative. In case of marked physiologic resorption, extraction is usually the treatment of choice.

Lateral luxation

Lateral luxation of primary teeth is the most common injury; and usually does not require treatment, as the crown is displaced lingually and the apex and cortical bone plate labially, i.e. away from the developing tooth germ. Unless occlusion dictates otherwise, a laterally luxated incisor can be left untreated. Over a period of 2-4 months, tongue pressure will reposition the tooth (Fig. 10.7).

In rare instances (e.g. after a fall with an object in the mouth), the laterally luxated tooth will be displaced in the opposite direction, i.e. with the apex forced into the follicle. In this case, extraction is the treatment of choice in order to prevent further damage to the permanent tooth germ.

Fig. 10.7. **Lateral luxation, repositioning indicated**
This 2-year-old boy suffered a lateral luxation. Due to occlusal interference, the tooth had to be repositioned. At a subsequent control, there is evidence of pulpal revascularization, as the root canal has become obliterated.

INJURIES TO THE PRIMARY DENTITION

Intrusion

Due to the labial tilt of primary incisor roots, most roots of intruded primary incisors will be forced through the labial bone plate as a result of an axial impact. Foreshortening of the intruded incisor in an occlusal radiographic exposure normally confirms this direction of displacement (Fig. 10.8). In such case, reeruption of the primary incisor should be anticipated and will normally occur within 2-4 months after injury (Fig. 10.9).

In the few cases where intrusive forces displace the primary incisor root into the follicle zone, removal of the displaced tooth is essential to relieve the pressure upon the odontogenic tissue within the follicle (Fig. 10.10).

When displacement of the primary incisor requires removal, it is essential that the extraction procedure does not elicit further injury to the developing permanent successor (Fig. 10.10). Therefore, it is necessary that certain guidelines are followed. Thus, because of the eminent risk of collision with the permanent tooth germ, elevators should never be used to luxate the primary incisor. Forceps should be the only instrument employed

Fig. 10.8. **Intrusion, the follicle not invaded**
This 4-year-old boy suffered intrusion of a central incisor. A lateral radiograph demonstrated no interference with the follicle. At later examination, reeruption of the intruded incisor is seen. There is no sign of pulp necrosis.

Fig. 10.9. Spontaneous re-eruption of an intruded primary incisor

This 2-year old boy suffered an intrusion of the right central incisor. The foreshortened radigraphic appearance of the intruded tooth implies labial displacement. Spontaneous re-eruption is therefore anticipated.

Follow-up, 2 months after injury

The tooth has erupted approximately 2 mm coronally.

Fullow-up, 3 months after injury

The tooth lacks 1 mm for complete eruption.

Follow-up, 1 year after injury

The tooth is in normal position. Crown color is normal and radiographs show no sign of pathology.

INJURIES TO THE PRIMARY DENTITION

Fig. 10.10. **Intrusion with severe follicle invasion**

This 1-year-old boy received an axial impact, resulting in complete intrusion of the central incisor. Note the displacement of the permanent tooth germ in the follicle. Removal of the primary incisor is mandatory.

Removing the displaced tooth

Using sedation and topical anesthesia, the tooth is grasped proximally with forceps and removed in a labial direction. The fractured and displaced palatal bone is repositioned with digital pressure and a suture placed to close the entrance to the socket.

Follow-up

At examination 1 week later, a slight change in the position of the tooth germ is seen.

Disturbancc in eruption

At the age of 6 years, it is evident that a crown dilaceration has developed.

150

for this purpose. Moreover, the primary incisor should be grasped by the proximal surfaces, as there is a risk that if the tooth is grasped faciolingually that the forceps could glide along the crown apically into the follicle zone. Once grasped mesiodistally, the displaced incisor should be lifted out of its socket in a labial and axial direction. Finally, once extracted, digital pressure should be applied to the buccal and lingual aspects of the socket to reposition the displaced bone plates. If necessary, a single suture should be used to approximate the facial and oral gingiva and thereby narrow the entrance to the socket.

In those cases where extraction is not indicated, one must be aware of the risk of infection due to impaction of bacterial plaque at the site of trauma. Signs of infection include swelling, spontaneous bleeding, abscess formation and fever. In these cases, the traumatized incisor must be removed and antibiotic therapy instituted (Fig. 10.11).

Fig. 10.11. Acute infection after intrusion
This 3-year-old boy suffered intrusion of two central incisors. As the root tips were displaced away from the developed tooth germ, spontaneous eruption was anticipated.

Follow-up, 2 weeks after injury
Acute infection with swelling and pus formation around the displaced incisors has developed necessitating extraction of both teeth.

151

INJURIES TO THE PRIMARY DENTITION

Avulsion

Replantation of avulsed primary teeth is contraindicated, as pulp necrosis is such a frequent event. Moreover, there is a risk of further injury to the permanent tooth germ by the replantation procedure whereby the coagulum can be forced into the area of the follicle.

Fig. 10.12. **Clinical and radiographic follow-up**
Reversal of coronal discoloration of a subluxated primary incisor.

Follow-up, 3 weeks after injury
Intense reddish brown discoloration is seen.

Follow-up, 1 year after injury
The color has changed to yellow and the radiographs demonstrate pulp canal obliteration.

Follow-up procedures

All traumas in the primary dentition resulting in displacement of the primary teeth (i.e. implying possible damage to the neurovascular supply) should be monitored, as infected pulp necrosis is a likely event, affecting approximately one third of all displaced teeth. A suggested follow-up schedule includes radiographic and clinical examination 1 and 2 months after injury (to ascertain spontaneous reeruption of the displaced tooth and early pulpal complications); and 1 year (to diagnose late pulpal complications as well as eventual malformation of the permanent successor).

With respect to pulp necrosis, it should be considered that reversible color changes of the crown are very frequent (Fig. 10. 12).

General prognosis

Data on the prognosis of traumatized primary teeth are scarce with respect to the risk of trauma to the developing permanent tooth germ. However, both age at time of injury and type of luxation appear to influence the permanent dentition (Figs. 10.13 and 10.14).

Fig. 10.13. **Risk of developmental disturbances in the permanent dentition according to the type of trauma** (after Andreasen & Ravn, 1970)

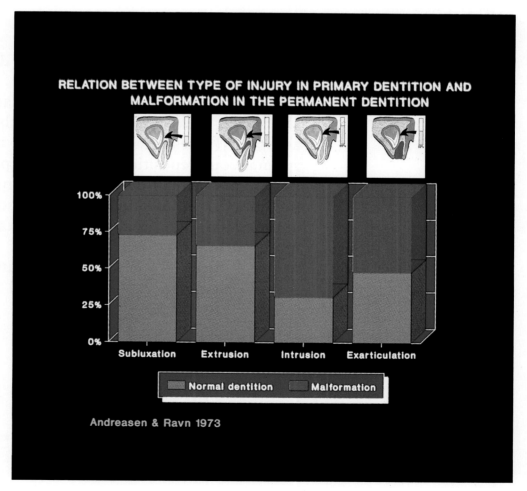

RELATION BETWEEN TYPE OF INJURY IN PRIMARY DENTITION AND MALFORMATION IN THE PERMANENT DENTITION

Subluxation Extrusion Intrusion Exarticulation

Normal dentition   Malformation

Andreasen & Ravn 1973

153

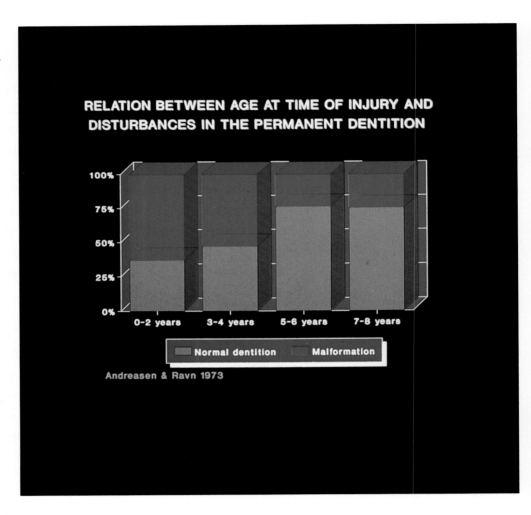

Fig. 10.14. **Risk of developmental disturbances in the permanent dentition according to the age of patient** (after Andreasen & Ravn, 1970)

Essentials

– Verify eventual collision between a displaced primary tooth and its permanent successor.
– If this has occurred, remove the displaced incisor.
– Otherwise, the displaced position of the luxated incisor can be accepted (unless it interferes with occlusal function); and spontaneous repositioning can be expected. With the conservative approach to dental trauma, one must be aware of the possible risk of infection due to impaction of bacterial plaque at the trauma site. In this case, the luxated incisor must also be removed.
– Monitor healing regularly with routine clinical and radiographic examinations (i.e. after 1 and 2 years).

Soft Tissue Injuries

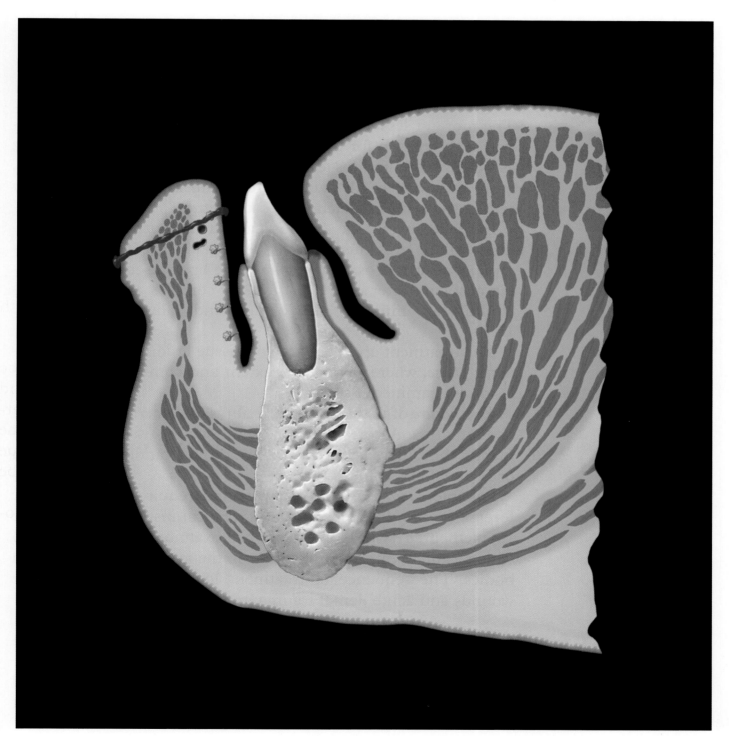

Pattern of injury and diagnosis

The more or less complete labial cover which shields the dentition is the reason for the large number of dental traumas being associated with injuries to the lip, gingiva and oral mucosa. Thus, more than half of all patients treated in a hospital emergency setting showed associated soft tissue injury.

In the following, the diagnosis and treatment of soft tissue injuries will be presented. The tissues usually involved are the gingiva, alveolar mucosa and the lips. The lips present specific healing problems after injury due to their complex anatomy that includes skin, mucosa, musculature and salivary glands (Fig. 11.1).

The treatment approach for soft tissue lesions includes a *diagnostic phase*, where the nature, extent and comtamination of the lesion is examined.

The *nature* of the injury can be abrasion, laceration, contusion or tissue loss. Ascertainment of the *extent* of tissue damage demands thorough exploration after administration of infiltration or regional block anesthesia.

Possible *contamination* of the wound requires inspection for foreign bodies. In deeper wounds, clinical inspection should be supplemented with a radiographic examination (see p. 164) which can reveal at least some of the contaminating foreign bodies. The sequence of treatment in the case of soft tissue wounds and acute dental trauma implies the following.

Initial treatment of dental injuries prior to soft tissue management

If reversed, the treatment of dental injuries (i.e. reposition and application of splints) may represent a hazard to the sutured soft tissue wounds.

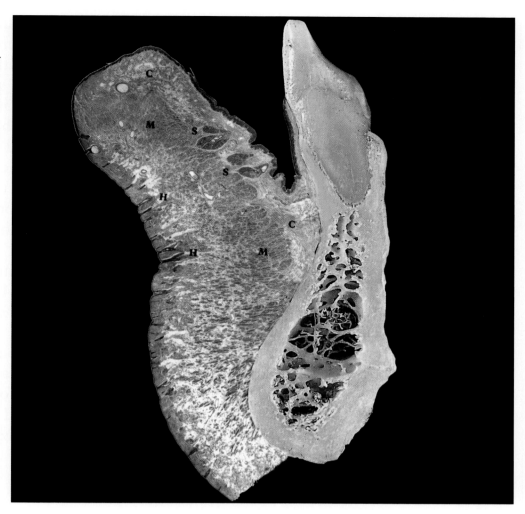

Fig. 11.1. **Section through a human lower lip in the midline**

Note the composite structure of the lip, with musculature, salivary glands and hair follicles. Most of the musculature is oriented parallel to the vermilion border. M = musculature, H = hair, C = connective tissue, S = salivary glands.

Wound cleansing and debridement

One of the aims of wound cleansing is to remove or neutralize microorganisms which contaminate the wound surface in order to prevent infection.

This implies removal of all foreign bodies and contused tissues as well as rinsing the lesion with saline.

Repositioning and suturing of displaced tissues

Based on the sparse clinical documentation it seems reasonable – until further studies are presented – to restrict the prophylactic use of antibiotics in soft tissue wounds to the following situations:

1. When the wound is heavily contaminated and wound debridement is not optimal (e.g. impacted foreign bodies or otherwise compromised wound cleansing).
2. When wound debridement has been delayed (i.e. more than 24 hours).
3. When the general defense system of the patient is compromised (e.g. diabetes, alcohol abuse, immunocompromised patients, patients with prosthetic heart valves or patients suffering from endocarditis).
4. Human or animal bite wounds.

If prophylactic antibiotic coverage is decided upon, early institution is very important. Thus, experimental studies have shown that the first 3 hours after trauma are critical; i.e. to obtain an optimal effect from the antibiotics, they should be administered within this period. If delayed, contaminating bacteria may multiply and invade the wound. Antibiotics should therefore be administered before surgery and maintained for 24 hours. The antibiotic of choice is Penicillin (Phenoxymethyl penicillin). The dosage (adults) should be: 2 million units (=1.2 g) p.o. at once followed by 2 million units (1.2 g) b.i.d. for 1 day. For children the dosage is 1 million units (0.6 g) p.o. at once followed by 1 million units (0.6 g) b.i.d. for 1 day.

In case of Penicillin allergy, Erythromycin should be administered. The dosage (adults) should be: 1 g p.o. at once followed by 1 g b.i.d. for 1 day. For children, the dosage is 0.5 g p.o. at once followed by 0.5 g b.i.d. for 1 day.

Tetanus prophylaxis should always be considered in the case of contaminated wounds. In case of a previously immunized patient (i.e. longer than 10 years previous to injury), a dose of 0.5 ml tetanus toxoid should be used (booster injection). In unimmunized patients, passive immunization should be provided.

Foreign Bodies

The presence of foreign bodies in the wound significantly increases the risk of infection and retards healing, even in wounds initially free of infection. This finding emphasizes the importance of adequate cleansing of the wound prior to suturing.

The removal of foreign bodies in facial and oral tissues after trauma is known to be a difficult and time-consuming procedure. A syringe with saline under high pressure, a scrub brush or gauze swabs soaked in saline can be used to remove foreign bodies. If this is not effective, a surgical blade (no. 11 or 15) or a small spoon escavator may be used (see p. 163). Complete removal of all foreign bodies is important, to prevent infection and also to prevent disfiguring scarring or tattooing.

Devitalized soft tissue serves to enhance infection by at least three mechanisms: First, as a culture medium that can promote bacterial growth; second, by inhibiting leukocyte migration, phagocytosis and subsequent bacterial kill; and third, by limiting leukocyte function due to the anaerobic environment within devitalized tissue.

For these reasons severely contused and/or ischemic tissue should be removed in order to facilitate healing.

Suturing

A general principle in wound treatment is the approximation of wound edges in order to reduce the distance for the wound healing module and thereby increase the speed of healing.

The tissue response to various types of sutures in the oral mucosa has been studied extensively in animals and in humans whereby a vigorous inflammatory reaction around the sutures could be demonstrated.

The general findings in these experimental studies have been that silk and catgut sutures (plain or chromic) elicited a very intense clinical and histological inflammatory reaction after 3, 5 and 7 days; whereas polyglycol acid (Dexon®) showed considerably less clinical and histological reaction.

The greatest part of the inflammatory reaction is probably related to the presence of bacteria within the interstices of multifilament suture materials. A further finding has been that monofilament sutures (e.g. nylon and Prolene®) display a significant reduction of adverse reactions compared to multifilament sutures, a finding possibly related to a reduced wick effect of monofilament sutures.

Finally, it should be borne in mind that it has been shown experimentally that there is an increased risk of infection with both increased suture diameter and submucosal/subcutaneous suture length.

The essential lesson of all these experiments in suturing and subsequent wound healing is therefore: use *a minimal number* of sutures with a *small diameter*, preferably *monofilament* and, finally, institute *early suture removal* (i.e. after 3-4 days in oral tissues), eventually in two stages, i.e. 3 and 6 days.

Treatment of Oral Soft Tissue Injuries

Gingival Wounds

The gingiva can present a variety of sequelae to frontal and horizontal impacts, such as abrasion, contusion or separation from the neck of the tooth.

Abrasion of the gingiva
Treatment can be limited to removal of any possible foreign bodies.

Laceration of the gingiva
After administration of a local anesthetic, the wound is cleansed with saline, and foreign bodies removed. The lacerated gingiva is brought back into normal position, implying that displaced teeth have been repositioned. After repositioning of the gingiva, the **159**

Fig. 11.2. Treatment of horizontal gingival laceration with tissue displacement in the permanent dentition
Due to an impact the gingiva has been lacerated and displaced whereas the central incisors are left intact.

Treatment
The displaced attached gingiva is repositioned and sutured.

necessary number of thin sutures (e.g. 5.0 or 6.0 silk or Prolene®) are placed to prevent displacement of tissue. In that regard, a minimum number of sutures should be used (Fig. 11.3). The patient is then placed on an oral hygiene regimen using 0.1% chlorhexidine for 4-5 days, whereafter the sutures are removed.

In case of trauma to the primary dentition, an impact often occurs parallel to the front of the maxilla or the mandible, which can result in complete displacement of the labial mucosa into the sulcus area (Fig 11.3). In these cases, it is necessary to reposition the gingiva, as exposure of the labial bone leads to protracted healing with subsequent gingival retraction and sometimes sequestration of the denuded labial bone. The same type of gingival displacement may also occur in the permanent dentition (Fig. 11.4).

With minor displacement or loss, gingival regeneration amounting to approximately 1 mm will usually occur.

Contusion of gingiva

In these cases, it is essential that optimal oral hygiene is maintained during the healing period. Due to the excellent vascularity in the area, revacularization of ischemic gingiva is often possible.

Fig. 11.3. Treatment of a gingival laceration with exposure of bone in the primary dentition

Due to a fall against an object, the gingiva has been displaced into the labial sulcus and bone is exposed whereas the incisors are left intact.

Repositioning and suturing of the gingiva

The condition immediately after gingival repositioning and suturing. Loose parts of the labial bone plate labial bone has been removed.

Fig. 11.4. Treatment of a vertical gingival laceration with tissue displacement in the permanent dentition

Due to an impact parallel to the front of the maxilla, the gingiva has been lacerated and displaced apically, whereas the incisors are left intact.

Treatment and follow-up

The displaced attached gingiva is repositioned and sutured.

161

SOFT TISSUE INJURIES

Lip Wounds

Skin or mucosal abrasion

If the direction of impact is parallel to the lip, the surface layer of the skin or the mucosa are peeled off and foreign bodies are often impressed into the wound. These foreign bodies are usually gravel or asphalt. Any failure to remove foreign bodies may lead to disfiguring scarring and discoloring (asphalt tattoo) (Fig. 11.5).

After administration of local anesthesia, the wound and surroundings are washed with a wound detergent (Fig. 11.6). Thereafter, all foreign bodies are removed with a small excavator

Fig. 11.6. **Treatment of a combined soft and hard tissue injury**
An 8-year-old girl has had a fall with her bike. She hit the ground with the lower part of her face. There is displacement of the right central incisor and laceration of the gingiva. The lips show extensive abrasions with asphalt deep in soft tissue wounds.

Cleaning the patient
The patient's face is washed with a mild wound detergent and the oral cavity rinsed with a water spray.

162

Rinsing the skin wounds
In order to adequately cleanse the abrasions, a topical anesthetic is necessary. In this case a Lidocain® spray was used. Note that the nostrils are compressed during the spraying procedure in order to reduce discomfort caused by spray entering the nose.

Washing the wounds
The lips are washed with surgical sponges or gauze sponges soaked in a mild disinfectant.

Removing asphalt particles
The impacted foreign bodies cannot be adequately removed by scrubbing or washing, but should be removed with a small excavator or a surgical blade kept perpendicular to the direction of the abrasions.

Follow-up
Two weeks after injury (right), the soft tissue wounds have healed without scarring.

SOFT TISSUE INJURIES

Fig. 11.7. **Split lip due to a frontal impact**
This patient was hit in the face with a bottle, resulting in a split lip and lateral luxation of the right central incisor. The vermilion border is sutured first, whereafter the rest of the laceration is closed with interrupted sutures (e.g. Prolene® 6.0).

or a surgical blade which is placed perpendicular to the cutaneous surface in order to prevent it from cutting into tissue. The wound is either left open or covered with a bandage.

Lip lacerations

Lip injuries are the result of a localized impact to the lips. Depending upon the angulation of impact, different types of lesions (split or penetrating lesions) will occur. In case of a frontal impact, the labial surfaces of protruding incisors may act as a bayonet, resulting in a sagittal split of the lip (Fig. 11.7). Due to the circumferential orientation of the orbicularis oris muscles, these wounds will usually gape, with initally intense arterial bleeding due to the rich vasculature in the region. Hemorrhage, however, is soon arrested due to vasoconstriction and coagulation.

If the direction of impact is parallel to the axis of either the maxillary or mandibular incisors, the incisal edges may penetrate the entire thickness of the lip (Fig. 11.8). When the incisal edges hit the impacting object, fracture of the tooth crown usually occurs. Upon retraction of the lip, foreign bodies such as tooth fragments, plaque, calculus and fragments from the impacting object usually become trapped within the lip.

Diagnosis and treatment

Diagnosis consists of determining the extent of the wound and verifying the presence of foreign bodies. In that regard, a radiographic examination will be able to demonstrate a variety of typical foreign bodies, such as tooth fragments, calculus, gravel, glass and fragments of paint (Fig. 11.9). However, other typical foreign bodies such as cloth and wood cannot be seen.

The radiographic technique consists of placing a dental film between the lip and the alveolar process. In case of a wide lesion, orientation of images is facilitated by placing a small metal indicator (e.g. a piece of lead foil) in the midline of the vermillion border in order to locate possible foreign bodies. The exposure should be made at a low kilovoltage (to increase contrast), and

164

Fig. 11.8. **Penetrating lip lesion with embedded foreign body**

This 8-year-old boy fell against a staircase, whereby the maxillary incisors penetrated the prolabium of the lower lip. Parallel lesions are found corresponding to each penetrating incisor.

Radiographic demonstration of foreign bodies

A dental film was placed between the lip and the dental arch. Exposure time is 1/4 of that for conventional dental radiographs. A large occlusal film is placed on the check and a lateral exposure taken using half the normal exposure time.

Radiographic demonstration of multiple foreign bodies in the lower lip

Orthoradial and lateral exposures show multiple fragments in lower lip. The lateral exposure could demonstrate that the fragments are equally distributed from the cutaneous to the mucosal aspect of the lip.

Retrieved dental fragments

The lip lesion is sutured after removal of tooth fragments.

165

the exposure time should be kept to approximately 25% of a usual dental exposure.

If the intraoral film discloses foreign bodies, a lateral exposure at 50% of the usual exposure time should be made in order to verify their position in a sagittal plane (Fig. 11.8).

Treatment of lip lesions should await completion of treatment of dental injuries (Fig. 11.10). A regional block anesthesia is administered (infiltration anesthesia of the wound may increase the risk of infection). Treatment starts by cleansing the wound and surrounding tissue with a wound detergent. The wound edges are elevated and foreign bodies are found and retrieved. It is essential to consider that foreign bodies are usually contained within small cul de sacs within the wound. When all fragments that have been registered radiographically have been retrieved, the wound is debrided for contused muscle and salivary gland tissue. Thereafter the wound is carefully rinsed with saline; and a check is made to ensure that bleeding has been arrested. The mucosal side of the wound is then sutured tightly so that no saliva can enter the wound. Thereafter, the cutaneous part of the wound is closed with fine sutures (e.g. 6.0 silk or Prolene®). Normally it is not necessary to use buried sutures, as the muscles along the wound edges will adapt to each other. Sutures placed in the musculature will induce scar formation because of their slow resorption and concomitant inflammation. Magnifying lenses, e.g. ordinary spectacles with 4 x loupes can be used to ensure meticulous suturing. The anatomy of the wound should be respected. Never excise wounds to make long straight scars which invariably are more visible.

In case of narrow penetrating wounds, a special technique of opening up the wound as illustrated in Fig. 11.11 is recommended.

Concerning the use of antibiotics, see p. 158.

CHAPTER 11

Fig. 11.10. Treatment of a broad penetrating lip lesion

Penetrating lesion of the upper lip in a 66-year-old woman due to a fall. Clinical appearance 4 hours after injury.

Dental injuries

The crown of the left central and lateral incisors and canine have been fractured while the lateral incisor and canine have been intruded. Soft tissue radiographs demonstrate two foreign bodies in the upper lip.

Wound cleansing

The cutaneous and mucosal aspects of the wounds are cleansed with a surgical detergent followed by saline.

Removal of foreign bodies

All radiographically demonstrated tooth fragments are located and removed.

Wound debridement

Traumatized salivary glands are excised in order to promote rapid healing.

Wound closure

The intraoral wound is closed with interrupted 4.0 silk sutures.

Repeated cleansing of the cutaneous wound

The cutaneous aspect of the wound is cleansed with saline to minimize contamination from closure of the mucosal wound.

Buried sutures

As a matter of principle, buried sutures should be kept to a minimum; and, when indicated, be resorbed over a short period of time (e.g. Vicryl® sutures). The point of entry of the needle should be remote from the oral and cutaneous wound surfaces in order to place the knot (i.e. the most infection-prone part of the suture) far from the wound edges; that is, at approximately one-half total thickness of the lip.

168

Assessing cutaneous wound closure

After closing the musclar tissue, the cutaneous part of the wound is evaluated. It is important that after muscular approximation, the wound edges can be approximated without tension. If this is not possible, approximation of the muscular part of the wound must be revised.

Suturing the cutaneous wound

Wound closure is principally begun at the vermilion border, the most critical part of the wound from an esthetic point. In cases where the wound is parallel to the vermilion border, the first suture is placed at a site where irregularities of the wound edge ensure an anatomically correct closure. The wound is closed with fine, monofilament interrupted sutures (Prolene® 6.0), under magnification (i.e. using spectacles with a 2 or 4 x magnification).

Suturing completed

The wound is now fully closed and antibiotics administered (i.e. penicillin, 1 million IU x 4, for 2 days).

Healing 6 weeks after injury

There is a minimum of scarring.

Fig. 11.11. Treatment of narrow penetrating lip lesion

This 27-year-old man fell, whereby the right central incisor penetrated the lower lip and fractured. Multiple tooth fragments are buried in the lip.

Removing foreign bodies from the lip

After administration of local anesthesia the narrow penetrating wound is opened using a pincette. When the pincette is open, a rectangular wound is formed whereby two sides of the wound become clearly visible. Foreign bodies are removed and the wound cleansed with saline.

Repeating the cleansing procedure

The pincette is turned 90° and the procedure is repeated.

Suturing the wound

The wound is sutured with interrupted 6.0 silk sutures. A radiograph shows that all fragments have been removed.

170

Essentials

Type of Soft Tissue Lesion
The type of lesion can be abrasion, laceration, contusion (including hematoma) or tissue loss (avulsion).

Treatment Principles include the following:
– Cleansing of the wound with a detergent.
– Repositioning of displaced tissues.
– Immobilization of the tissue, usually with sutures.

Gingival Wounds (Figs. 11.2 to 11.4)
a. Rinse the wound and surroundings with a wound detergent.
b. Reposition displaced gingiva.
c. Place a few fine sutures.
d. Instruct in good oral hygiene including daily mouth rinse with 0.1% chlorhexidine.
e. Remove sutures after 4-5 days.

Lip Wounds

Skin or Mucosal Abrasions (Fig. 11.6)

Split Lip Wounds (Fig. 11.7)
Use the same procedure as for penetrating lip lesions. However, in this case a few buried resorbable sutures are indicated (e.g. Dexon® 4.0/5.0).

Penetrating Lip Wounds (Figs. 11.8 to 11.11)
a. Administer antibiotics if indicated.
b. Take a radiograph of the lip. (Use 25% of the normal exposure time).
c. Use a regional anesthesia.
d. Rinse the wound and surroundings with a wound detergent.
e. Remove foreign bodies and contused muscle and salivary gland tissue.
f. Suture the labial mucosa first.
g. Rinse the wound again with saline.
h. Suture the cutaneous wound with fine sutures (6.0 nylon or Prolene®).
i. Remove sutures after 4-5 days.

Appendix 1

Emergency record for acute dental trauma

Patient's name Birthdate	

Date of examination: Time of examination:	Referred by: Referring diagnosis:

General medical history: any serious illness?   [yes] [no]
If yes, explain.

Previous dental injuries?   [yes] [no]
If yes,
   When?
   Which teeth were injured?
   Treatment given and by whom?

Present dental injury:
   Date: Time:
   Where?
   How?

Have you had or have now *headache?*   [yes] [no]

Have you had or have now *nausea?*   [yes] [no]

Have you had or have now *vomiting?*   [yes] [no]

Were you *unconscious* at the time of injury?   [yes] [no]
If yes, for how long (minutes)?
Can you *remember* what happened before,   [yes] [no]
during or after the accident?

The emergency record is constructed so that wherever a question is answered by *yes*, more details must be provided. Finally, the last question in the record is whether the examiner has re-read the chart. This is a reminder to check that all relevant points have been registered.

173

Emergency record for acute dental trauma

Is there pain from *cold air?* `yes` `no`
If yes, *which teeth?*

Is there pain or tenderness from *occlusion?* `yes` `no`
If yes, *which teeth?*

Constant pain? `yes` `no`
If yes, *which teeth?*

Treatment elsewhere? `yes` `no`
If yes, *what treatment?*

After *exarticulation,* the following information is needed:
Where were the teeth found (dirt, asphalt, floor, etc.)?
When were the teeth found?
Were the teeth *dirty?*
How were the teeth *stored?*
Were the teeth *rinsed* and *with what* prior to replantation?
When were the teeth replanted?
Was *tetanus toxoid* given?
Were *antibiotics* given?
   Antibiotic?
   Dosage?

Objective examination
Is the patient's general condition affected? `yes` `no`
If yes, *pulse*
       blood pressure
       pupillary reflex
       cerebral condition
Objective findings beyond the head and neck? `yes` `no`
If yes, *type* and *location*
Objective findings within the head and neck? `yes` `no`
If yes, *type* and *location*

174

APPENDIX 1

Emergency record for acute dental trauma

Objective examination – Extraoral findings (contd.)		
Bleeding from nose, or rhinitis	yes	no
Bleeding from ext. auditory canal	yes	no
Double vision or limited eye movement	yes	no
Palpable signs of fracture of facial skeleton	yes	no
If yes, *location of fracture*		

Objective examination – Intraoral findings		
Lesions of the *oral mucosa*	yes	no
If yes, *type* and *location*		
Gingival lesion	yes	no
If yes, *type* and *location*		
Tooth fracture	yes	no
If yes, *type* and *location*		
Alveolar fracture	yes	no
If yes, *type* and *location*		

Supplemental information:

General condition of the dentition			
Caries	poor	fair	good
Periodontal status	poor	fair	good
Horizontal occlusal relationship	undr bite	over jet	norm
Vertical occlusal relationship	deep	open	norm

Radiographic findings
Tooth dislocation
Root fracture
Bone fracture
Pulp canal obliteration
Root resorption

Photographic registration		
	yes	no

175

Emergency record for acute dental trauma

Diagnoses (check appropriate boxes and designate tooth no. or indicate correct anatomical region)

☐ Infraction

☐ Complicated crown fracture

☐ Uncomplicated crown fracture

☐ Complicated crown-root fracture

☐ Uncomplicated crown-root fracture

☐ Root Fracture

☐ Alveolar fracture

☐ Mandibular fracture

☐ Maxillary fracture

☐ Concussion

☐ Subluxation

☐ Extrusion

☐ Lateral luxation

☐ Intrusion

☐ Exarticulation

☐ Skin abrasion

☐ Skin laceration

☐ Skin contusion

☐ Mucosal abrasion

☐ Mucosal laceration

☐ Mucosal contusion

☐ Gingival abrasion

☐ Gingival laceration

☐ Gingival contusion

Supplementary remarks:

Treatment plan
At time of injury: *Final therapy:*
Repositioning (time finished)
Fixation (time finished)
Pulpal therapy (time finished)
Dentinal coverage (time finished)

Chart re-read by examining dentist   ☐ yes   ☐ no

Appendix 2

Clinical examination form for the time of injury and follow-up examinations

	Tooth no.	12		11		21		22	
T I M E O F I N J U R Y	Date								

	Tooth color
	   normal
	   yellow
	   red
	   grey
	   crown restoration								

	Displacement (mm)
	   intruded
	   extruded
	   protruded
	   retruded								

	Loosening (0-3)								
	Tenderness to percussion ($+/-$)								
	Pulp test (value)								
	Ankylosis tone ($+/-$)								
	Occlusal contact ($+/-$)								
C O N T R O L	Fistula ($+/-$)								
	Gingivitis ($+/-$)								
	Gingival retraction (mm)								
	Abnormal pocketing ($+/-$)								

Each column represents an examination of a given tooth. The first column for each tooth gives the values from the time of injury. *Only* the parameters listed in the top half of the form ("Time of injury") are to be recorded at the time of injury. The information from this examination as well as the information collected on the emergency record are used to determine the final diagnoses for the injured teeth. Those parameters *and* the last four (fistula, gingivitis, gingival retraction, abnormal pocketing) are to be registered at all follow-up controls.

Appendix 3

Clinical and radiographic findings with the various luxation types

Findings	Concussion	Subluxation	Extrusion	Lateral Luxation	Intrusion
Clinical					
Abnormal mobility	−	+	+	−(+)	−(+)
Tenderness to percussion	+	+(−)*	+/−	−(+)	−(+)
Percussion sound**	normal	dull	dull	metallic	metallic
Response to pulp testing	+/−	+/−	−(+)	−(+)	−(+)
Clinical dislocation	−	−	+	+	+
Radiographic dislocation	−	−	+	+	+

 * A sign in parentheses indicates a finding of rare occurrence.
** Teeth with incomplete root formation and teeth with marginal or periapical inflammatory lesions will also elicit a dull percussion sound.

178

Appendix 4

Summary of treatment and follow-up procedures and recall schedule following the various trauma types

Post-traumatic interval*	Radiographic exposure for various trauma types		
	Luxation of 21**	Replantation of 21	Root fracture of 21
Time of injury	OI 11,21*** BI 12,11,21,22	OI 11,21 BI 12,11,21,22	OI 11,21 BI 12,11,21,22
1 week		BI 21,22£$	
2-3 weeks	OI 11,21£$	BI 21,22	OI 11,21
6-8 weeks	BI 12,11,21,22£	BI 12,11,21,22	BI 12,11,21,22
3 months		BI 21,22	BI 12,11,21,22£
6 months		BI 21,22	
1 year	BI 12,11,21,22	BI 12,11,21,22	BI 12,11,21,22
2, 3, 4 years		BI 21,22	
5, 10, 15 years	BI 12,11,21,22	BI 12,11,21,22	BI 12,11,21,22

    * All examinations include radiographs as well as information from the clinical examination form (see Appendix 2).

   ** Tooth designation is according to the FDI two-digit system.

 *** Regarding radiographic exposure, OI implies "Occlusal Identical", or occlusal exposures; BI implies "bisecting identical". Both designations imply the use of standardized techniques and filmholder.

£ Removal of fixation. The following fixation periods are suggested. The reader is referred to the respective chapters for details: Replantation, 1 week; Extrusion, 2-3 weeks; Lateral luxation, 3-8 weeks (depending on radiographic findings); Intrusion, see text for discussion of repositioning and fixation; Root fracture, 3 months.

$ Begin endodontic therapy: Replantation, after 1 week, Intrusion, after 2 weeks.

179

Bibliography

Chapter 1. Examination of the patient, wound healing and treatment principles

1. ANDREASEN JO, ANDREASEN FM. Classification, etiology and epidemiology of traumatic dental injuries. In: ANDREASEN JO, ANDREASEN FM. *Textbook and Color Atlas of Traumatic injuries to the Teeth*. 3rd. ed. Copenhagen: Munksgaard Publishers, 1994; p. 151-177.
2. ANDREASEN FM, ANDREASEN JO. Diagnosis of luxation injuries. The importance of standardized clinical, radiographic and photographic techniques in clinical investigations. *Endod Dent Traumatol* 1985; 1: 160-9.
3. ANDREASEN JO. Etiology and pathogenesis of traumatic dental injuries. A clinical study of 1,289 cases. *Scand J Dent Res* 1970; 78: 329-42.
4. ANDREASEN JO, RAVN JJ. Epidemiology of traumatic dental injuries to primary and permanent teeth in a Danish population sample. *Int J Oral Surg* 1972; 1: 235-9.
5. *Application of the International Classification of Diseases to Dentistry and Stomatology*. IDC-DA 3rd ed. Geneva: WHO, 1995.
6. BAKLAND LK, ANDREASEN JO. Examination of the dentally traumatized patient. *Calif Dent Ass J* 1996; 24: 35-44.
7. KOPEL HM, JOHNSON R. Examination and neurologic assessment of children with orofacial trauma. *Endod Dent Traumatol* 1985; 1: 155-159.
8. RAVN JJ. Dental injuries in Copenhagen schoolchildren, school years 1967-1972. *Communiti Dent Oral Epidemiol* 1974; 2: 231-45.
9. GOTTRUP F, ANDREASEN JO. Wound healing subsequent to injury. In: Andreasen JO, Andreasen FM. *Textbook and Color Atlas of Traumatic Injuries to the Teeth*. 3rd ed. Copenhagen; Munksgaard Publishers, 1993: p. 13-76.
10. ANDREASEN JO, TORABINEJAD M, FINKELMAN RD. Response of oral tissues to trauma and inflammation and mediators of hard tissue resorption. In: Andreasen JO, Andreasen FM. *Textbook and Color Atlas of Traumatic Injuries to the Teeth*. 3rd ed. Copenhagen; Munksgaard Publishers, 1993: p. 77-133.
11. ANDREASEN JO. External root resorption: its implication in dental traumatology, paedodontics, periodontics, orthodontics and endodontics. *Int Endod J* 1985: 18: 109-118.
12. ANDREASEN JO. Experimental dental traumatology: development of a model for external root resorption. *Endod Dent Traumatol* 1987, 3: 269-287.
13. ANDREASEN JO. Review of root resorption systems and models. Etiology of root resorption and the homeostatic mechanisms of the periodontal ligament. In: Davidovitch D, Ed. *The Biological Mechanisms of Tooth Eruption and Root Resorption*. Birmingham; EBSCO Media: 9-21.
14. ANDREASEN JO, ANDREASEN FM. Root resorption following traumatic dental injuries. *Proc Finn Dent Soc* 1991; 88: 95-114.

Chapter 2. Crown fracture

1. ANDREASEN JO, ANDREASEN FM. Crown fractures. In: ANDREASEN JO, ANDREASEN FM. *Textbook and Color Atlas of Traumatic Injuries to the Teeth*. 3rd ed. Copenhagen: Munksgaard Publishers, 1994; 219-250.
2. ANDREASEN FM, RINDUM JL, MUNKSGAARD EC, ANDREASEN JO. Bonding of enamel-dentin crown fractures with GLUMA® and resin. *Endod Dent Traumatol* 1986; 2: 277-80.
3. ANDREASEN FM, NORÉN JG, ANDREASEN JO, ENGELHARDTSEN S, LINDH-STRÖMBERG U. Long-term survival of crown fragment bonding in the treatment of crown fractures. A multicenter clinical study of fragment retention. *Quintessence Int* 1995; 26: 669-681.
4. BRÄNNSTRÖM M. Observations on exposed dentine and the corresponding pulp tissue. A preliminary study with replica and routine histology. *Odontol Revy* 1962; 13: 235-45.
5. CVEK M. A clinical report on partial pulpotomy and capping with calcium hydroxide in permanent incisors with complicated crown fracture. *J Endod* 1978; 4: 232-7.
6. CVEK M, LUNDBERG M. Histological appearance of pulps after exposure by a crown fracture, partial pulpotomy, and clinical diagnosis of healing. *J Endod* 1983; 9: 8-11.
7. CVEK M. Partial pulpotomy in crown-fractured incisors – Results 3 to 15 years after treatment. *Acta Stomatologica Croatica* 1993; 27: 167-73.
8. FARIK B, KREIBORG S, ANDREASEN JO. Adhesive bonding of fragmented anterior teeth. *Endod Dent Traumatol* 1998; 14: 199-123.
9. FUKS AB, CHOSACK A, KLEIN H, EIDELMAN E. Partial pulpotomy as a treatment alternative for exposed pulps in crown-fractured permanent incisors. *Endod Dent Traumatol* 1987; 3: 100-2.
10. GOLDBERG F, MASSONE EJ, SPIELBERG C. Evaluation of the dentinal bridge after pulpotomy and calcium hydroxide dressing. *J Endod* 1984; 10: 318-20.
11. HALLET GEM, PORTEOUS JR. Fractured incisors treated by vital pulpotomy. A report on 100 consecutive cases. *Br Dent J* 1963; 115: 279-87.
12. HELLE A, SIRKKANEN R, EVALAHTI M. Repair of fractured incisal edges with UV-light polymerized and self-polymerizing fissure sealants and composite resins. Two year report of 93 cases. *Proc Finn Dent Soc* 1975; 71: 87-90.
13. HOLLAND R, DE SOUZA, V, DE MELLO W, NERY MJ, BERNABE PFE, FILHO JAO. Permeability of the hard tissue bridge formed after pulpotomy with calcium hydroxide: a histologic study. *J Am Dent Assoc* 1979; 99: 472-5.
14. KOCH G, PAULANDER J. Klinisk uppföljning av compositrestaureringar utförda med emaljetsningsmetodik. *Swed Dent J* 1976; 69: 191-6.
15. LIM KC, KIRK EEJ. Direct pulp capping: a review. *Endod Dent Traumatol* 1987; 3: 213-9.

181

16. MADER C. Restoration of a fractured anterior tooth. *J Am Dent Assoc* 1978; 96: 113-5.
17. OLGART L, BRÄNNSTRÖM M, JOHNSON G. Invasion of bacteria into dentinal tubules. Experiments in vivo and in vitro. *Acta Odontol Scand* 1974; 32: 61-70.
18. RAVN JJ. Follow-up study of permanent incisors with enamel cracks as a result of an acute trauma. *Scand J Dent Res* 1981; 89: 117-22.
19. RAVN JJ. Follow-up study of permanent incisors with enamel fractures as a result of an acute trauma. *Scand J Dent Res* 1981; 89: 213-7.
20. RAVN JJ. Follow-up study of permanent incisors with enamel-dentin fractures after acute trauma. *Scand J Dent Res* 1981; 89: 355-65.
21. RAVN JJ. Follow-up study of permanent incisors with complicated crown fractures after acute trauma. *Scand J Dent Res* 1982; 90: 363-72.
22. ROBERTSON A, ANDREASEN FM, ANDREASEN JO, NORÉN JG, Prognosis of crown fractures with and without periodontal injury. 1999: In preparation.
23. SMALES RJ. Incisal angle adhesive restorations: a two-year clinical survey of three materials. *Australian Dent J* 1977; 22: 267-71.
24. SIMONSEN RJ. Restoration of a fractured central incisor using original tooth fragment. *J Am Dent Assoc* 1982; 105: 648-50.
25. TZIAFAS D, BELTES P. Pulp capping with calcium hydroxide: diagnostic value of radiographic findings. *Endod Dent Traumatol* 1988; 4: 260-4.
26. QVIST V, STRÖM C, THYLSTRUP A. Two-year assessment of anterior resin restorations inserted with two acid-etch restorative procedures. *Scand J Dent Res* 1985; 93: 343-50.

Chapter 3. Crown-root fracture

1. ANDREASEN FM, ANDREASEN JO. Crown-root fractures. In: ANDREASEN JO, ANDREASEN FM. *Textbook and Color Atlas of Traumatic Injuries to the Teeth* 3rd ed. Copenhagen: Munksgaard Publishers, 1993: 257-276.
2. HEITHERSAY GS. Combined endodontic-orthodontic treatment of transverse root fractures in the region of the alveolar crest. *Oral Surg Oral Med Oral Pathol* 1973; 36: 404-15.
3. INGBER JS. Forced eruption: Part II. A method of treatment nonrestorable teeth – periodontal and restorative considerations. *J Periodont* 1976; 47: 203-16.
4. KAHNBERG K-E, WARFVINGE J, BIRGERSSON B. Intraalveolar transplantation (I). The use of autologous bone transplants in the periapical region. *Int J Oral Surg* 1982; 11: 372-79.
5. KAHNBERG K-E. Intraalveolar transplantation of teeth with crown-root fractures. *J Oral Surg* 1985; 43: 38-42.
6. KAHNBERG K-E. Surgical extrusion of root-fractured teeth – A follow-up study of two surgical methods. *Endod Dent Traumatol* 1988; 4: 85-89.
7. TEGSJÖ U, VALERIUS-OLSSON H, OLGART K. Intra-alveolar transplantation of teeth with cervical root fractures. *Swed Dent J* 1978; 2: 73-82.
8. WARFVINGE, J. KAHNBERG K-E. Intraalveolar transplantation of teeth. IV. Endodontic considerations. *Swed Dent J* 1989; 13: 229-33.

Chapter 4. Root fracture

1. ANDREASEN FM, ANDREASEN JO. Root fractures. In: ANDREASEN JO, ANDREASEN FM. *Textbook and Color Atlas of Traumatic Injuries to the Teeth*. 3rd ed. Copenhagen: Munksgaard Publishers, 1993: 279-311.
2. ANDREASEN FM, ANDREASEN JO, BAYER T. Prognosis of root fractured permanent incisors – prediction of healing modalities. *Endod Dent Traumatol* 1989; 5: 11-22.
3. ANDREASEN FM, ANDREASEN JO. Resorption and mineralization processes following root fracture of permanent incisors. *Endod Dent Traumatol* 1988; 4: 202-14.
4. CVEK M. Treatment of non-vital permanent incisors with calcium hydroxide. IV. Periodontal healing and closure of the root canal in the coronal fragment of teeth with intraalveolar fracture and vital apical fragment. *Odontol Revy* 1974; 25: 239-45.
5. JACOBSEN I, ZACHRISSON BU. Repair characteristics of root fractures in permanent anterior teeth. *Scand J Dent Res* 1975; 83: 355-64.
6. JACOBSEN I. Root fractures in permanent anterior teeth with incomplete root formation. *Scand J Dent Res* 1976; 84: 210-7.
7. ZACHRISSON BU, JACOBSEN I. Long-term prognosis of 66 permanent anterior teeth with root fracture. *Scand J Dent Res* 1975; 83: 345-54.
8. RAVN JJ. En klinisk og radiologisk undersøgelse af 55 rodfrakturer i unge permanente incisiver. *Tandlægebladet* 1976; 80: 391-6.

Chapter 5. Concussion and subluxation

1. ANDREASEN FM, ANDREASEN JO. Luxation injuries. In: ANDREASEN JO, ANDREASEN FM. *Textbook and Color Atlas of Traumatic Injuries to the Teeth* 3rd ed. Copenhagen: Munksgaard Publishers, 1993: 315-82.
2. ANDREASEN FM, VESTERGAARD PEDERSEN B. Prognosis of luxated permanent teeth – the development of pulp necrosis. *Endod Dent Traumatol* 1985; 1: 207-20.
3. ANDREASEN FM. *Pulpal healing after luxation injuries and root fracture in the permanent dentition*. Thesis, Copenhaven University 1995. ISBN no. 87-985538-0-1.
4. EKLUND G, STÅLHANE I, HEDEGÅRD B. Traumatized permanent teeth in children aged 7-15 years. III. A multivariate analysis of posttraumatic complications of subluxated and luxated teeth. *Swed Dent J* 1976; 69: 179-89.
5. ROCK WP, GORDON PH, FRIEND LA, GRUNDY MC. The relationship between trauma and pulp death in incisor teeth. *Br Dent J* 1974; 136: 236-9.
6. STÅLHANE I, HEDEGÅRD B. Traumatized permanent teeth in children aged 7-15 years. Part II. *Swed Dent J* 1975; 68: 157-69.

Chapter 6. Extrusion and lateral luxation

1. ANDREASEN FM, ANDREASEN JO. Luxation injuries. In: ANDREASEN JO, ANDREASEN FM. *Textbook and Color Atlas of Traumatic Injuries to the Teeth* 3rd ed. Copenhagen: Munksgaard Publishers, 1994: 315-78.

2. ANDREASEN JO. Luxation of permanent teeth due to trauma. A clinical and radiographic follow-up study of 189 injured teeth. *Scand J Dent Res* 1970; 78: 273-86.
3. ANDREASEN FM, VESTERGAARD PEDERSEN B. Prognosis of luxated permanent teeth – the development of pulp necrosis. *Endod Dent Traumatol* 1985; 1: 207-20.
4. ANDREASEN FM, YU Z, THOMSEN BL. The relationship between pulpal dimensions and the development of pulp necrosis after luxation injuries in the permanent dention. *Endod Dent Traumatol* 1986; 2: 90-8.
5. ANDREASEN FM. Transient apical breakdown and its relation to color and sensibility changes. *Endod Dent Traumatol* 1986; 2: 9-19.
6. ANDREASEN FM. Histological and bacteriological study of pulps extirpated after luxation injuries. *Endod Dent Traumatol* 1988; 4: 170-81.
7. ANDREASEN FM, YU Z, THOMSEN BL, ANDERSEN PK. The occurrence of pulp canal obliteration after luxation injuries in the permanent dentition. *Endod Dent Traumatol* 1978; 3: 103-115.
8. ANDREASEN FM. Pulpal healing after luxation injuries and root fracture is the permanent dentition. *Endod Dent Traumatol* 1989; 5: 111-131.
9. DUMSHA T, HOVLAND EJ. Pulpal prognosis following extrusive luxation injuries in permanent teeth with closed apexes. *J Am Dent Assoc* 1982; 36: 410-2.
10. HERFORTH M. *Traumatische Schädigungen der Frontzähne bei Kindern und Jugendlichen im Alter von 7 bis 15 Jahren.* Berlin: Quintessenz Verlags-GmbH. 1982.
11. OIKARINEN K. Functional fixation for traumatically luxated teeth. *Endod Dent Traumatol* 1987; 3: 224-8.
12. OIKARINEN K, GUNDLACH KKH, PFEIFER G. Late complications of luxation injuries to teeth. *Endod Dent Traumatol* 1987; 3: 296-303.
13. ROCK WP, GRUNDY MC. The effect of luxation and subluxation upon the prognosis of traumatized incisor teeth. *J Dent* 1981; 9: 224-30.

Chapter 7. Intrusion

1. ANDREASEN FM, ANDREASEN JO. Luxation injuries. In: ANDREASEN JO, ANDREASEN FM. *Textbook and Color Atlas of Traumatic Injuries to the Teeth* 3rd ed. Copenhagen: Munksgaard Publishers, 1993: 315-82.
2. ANDREASEN FM. *Pulpal healing after luxation injuries and root fracture in the permanent dentition.* Thesis, Copenhagen University 1995. ISBN no. 87-985538-0-1.
3. ANDREASEN JO. Luxation of permanent teeth due to trauma. A clinical and radiographic follow-up study of 189 injured teeth. *Scand J Dent Res* 1970; 78: 273-86.
4. ANDREASEN FM, YU Z, THOMSEN BL. The relationship between dimensions and the development of pulp necrosis after luxation injuries in the permanent dentition. *Endod Dent Traumatol* 1986; 2: 90-8.
5. ANDREASEN FM, VESTERGAARD PEDERSEN B. Prognosis of luxation permanent teeth – the development of pulp necrosis. *Endod Dent Traumatol* 1985; 1: 207-20.

Chapter 8. Avulsion

1. ANDERSSON L, BODIN I, SÖRENSEN S. Progression of root resorption following replantation of human teeth after extended extra-oral storage. *Endod Dent Traumatol* 1989; 5: 38-47.
2. ANDERSSON L, BLOMLÖF L, LINDSKOG S, FEIGLIN B, HAMMARSTRÖM L. Tooth ankylosis. Clinical, radiographic and histological assessments. *Int J Oral Surg* 1984; 13: 423-31.
3. ANDREASEN JO, ANDREASEN FM. Avulsions, In: ANDREASEN JO, ANDREASEN FM. *Textbook and Color Atlas of Traumatic Injuries to the Teeth* 3rd ed. Copenhagen: Munksgaard Publishers, 1993: 383-420.
4. ANDREASEN JO. Replantation of avulsed teeth. In: ANDREASEN JO. *Atlas of Replantation and Transplantation of Teeth.* Freiburg: Mediglobe 1992: 57-97.
5. ANDREASEN JO, HJØRTING-HANSEN E. Replantation of teeth. I. Radiographic and clinical study of 110 human teeth replanted after accidental loss. *Acta Odontol Scand* 1966; 24: 263-86.
6. ANDREASEN JO, HJØRTING-HANSEN E. Replantation of teeth. II. Histological study of 22 replanted anterior teeth in humans. *Acta Odontol Scand* 1966; 24: 287-306.
7. ANDREASEN JO. Periodontal healing after replantation of traumatically avulsed human teeth. Assessment by mobility testing and radiography. *Acta Odontol Scand* 1975; 33: 325-35.
8. ANDREASEN JO, BORUM M, JACOBSEN HL, ANDREASEN FM. Replantation of 400 traumatically avulsed permanent incisors. I. Diagnosis of healing complications. *Endod Dent Traumatol* 1995; 11: 51-58.
9. ANDREASEN JO, BORUM M, JACOBSEN HL, ANDREASEN FM. Replantation of 400 avulsed permanent incisors. II. Factors related to pulp healing. *Endod Dent Traumatol* 1995; 11: 59-68.
10. ANDREASEN JO, BORUM M, ANDREASEN FM. Replantation of 400 avulsed permanent incisors. III. Factors related to root growth after replantation. *Endod Dent Traumatol* 1995; 11: 69-75.
11. ANDREASEN JO, BORUM M, JACOBSEN HL, ANDREASEN FM. Replantation of 400 avulsed permanent incisors. IV. Factors related to periodontal ligament healing. *Endod Dent Traumatol* 1995; 11: 76-89.
12. ANDREASEN JO, BORUM M, ANDREASEN FM. Progression of root resorption after replantation of 400 avulsed human incisors. In: Davidovitch Z (ed.) *The Biological Mechanisms of Tooth Eruption, Resorption and Replacement by Implants.* Boston: Harvard Society for the Advancement of Orthodontics, 1994. pp 577-582.
13. ANDREASEN JO. Periodontal healing after replantation of traumatically avulsed human teeth. Assessment by mobility testing and radiography. *Acta Odontol Scand* 1975; 33: 325-335.
14. AAE. Treatment of the avulsed permanent tooth. Recommended Guidelines of the American Association of Endodontists 1995.
15. BARRETT EJ, KENNY DJ. Avulsed permanent teeth: a review of the literature and treatment guidelines. *Endod Dent Traumatol* 1997; 13: 153-163.
16. COCCIA CT. A clinical investigation of root

183

resorption rates in reimplanted young permanent incisors: A five-year study. *J Endod* 1980; 6: 413-20.

17. CVEK M, GRANATH L-E, HOLLENDER L. Treatment of non-vital permanent incisors with calcium hydroxide. III. Variation of occurrence of ankylosis of reimplanted teeth with duration of extra-alveolar period and storage environment. *Odontol Revy* 1974; 25: 43-56.

18. GREGG TA, BOYD DH. UK National Clinical Guidelines in Paediatric Dentistry. Treatment of avulsed permanent teeth in children. *Int J Paediatric Dent* 1998; 8: 51-58.

19. HAMMARSTRÖM L, PIERCE A, BLOMLÖF L, FEIGLIN B, LINDSKOG S. Tooth avulsion and replantation – A review. *Endod Dent Traumatol* 1986; 2: 1-8.

20. KLING M, CVEK M, MEJARE I. Rate and predictability of pulp revascularization in therapeutically reimplanted permanent incisors. *Endod Dent Traumatol* 1986; 2: 83-89.

21. TROPE M, FRIEDMAN S. Periodontal healing of replanted dog teeth stored in Viaspan, milk and Hank's balanced salt solution. *Endod Dent Traumatol* 1992; 8: 183-88.

Chapter 9. Fractures of the alveolar process

1. ANDREASEN JO. Injuries to the supporting bone. In: ANDREASEN JO, ANDREASEN FM. *Textbook and Color Atlas of Traumatic Injuries to the Teeth*. 3rd ed. Copenhagen: Munksgaard Publishers, 1993: 427-53.

2. ANDREASEN JO. Fractures of the alveolar process of the jaw. A clinical and radiographic follow-up study. *Scand J Dent Res* 1970; 78: 263-72.

3. FREIHOFER HPM. Ergebnisse der Behandlung vom Alveolarforsatzfrakturen. *Schweiz Monatsschr Zahnheilk* 1969; 79: 623-29.

Chapter 10. Injuries to the primary dentition

1. ANDREASEN JO. Injuries to developing teeth. In. ANDREASEN JO, ANDREASEN FM. *Textbook and Color Atlas of Traumatic Injuries to the Teeth* 3rd ed. Copenhagen: Munksgaard Publishers, 1993: 459-491.

2. ANDREASEN JO, RAVN JJ. The effect of traumatic injuries to primary teeth on their permanent successors. II. A clinical and radiographic follow-up study of 213 injured teeth. *Scand J Dent Res* 1970; 79: 284-94.

3. ANDREASEN JO, RAVN JJ. Enamel changes in permanent teeth after trauma to their predecessors. *Scand J Dent Res* 1973; 81: 203-9.

4. ANDREASEN JO, SUNDSTRØM B, RAVN JJ. The effect of traumatic injuries to primary teeth on their permanent successors. I. A clinical, radiographic, microradiographic and electronmicrosopic study of 117 injured permanent teeth. *Scand J Dent Res* 1970; 79: 219-83.

5. BASSAT YB, BRIN I, FUKS A, ZILBERMAN Y. Effect of trauma to the primary incisors on permanent successors in different developmental stages. *Pediatric Dentistry* 1985; 7: 37-40.

6. DYNESEN H, RAVN JJ. Rodfrakturer i det primære tandsæt. *Tandlægebladet* 1973; 77: 865-8.

7. LIND V, WALLIN H, EGERMARK-ERIKSSON I, BERNHOLD M. Indirekta traumaskador. Kli-

niska skador på permanenta incisiver som följd av trauma mot temporära incisiver. *Sv Tandläkforb Tid* 1970; 62: 738-56.

8. RAVN JJ. Sequelae of acute mechanical traumata in the primary dentition. *ASDC J Dent Child* 1968; 35: 281-9.

9. RAVN JJ. Developmental disturbances in permanent teeth after exarticulation of their primary predecessors. *Scand J Dent Res* 1975; 83: 131-4.

10. RAVN JJ. Developmental disturbances in permanent teeth after intrusion of their primary predecessors. *Scand J Dent Res* 1976; 84: 137-41.

11. SELLISETH N-E. The significance of traumatised primary incisors on the development and eruption of permanent teeth. *Trans Eur Orthod Soc* 1970; 46: 443-59.

12. ZILBERMAN Y, FUKS A, BASSAT YB, BRIN I, LUSTMANN J. Effect of trauma to primary incisors on root development of their permanent successors. *Pediatric Dentistry* 1986; 4: 289-293.

Chapter 11. Soft tissue injuries

1. ANDREASEN JO. Soft tissue injuries. In: ANDREASEN JO, ANDREASEN FM. *Textbook and Colar Atlas of Traumatic Injuries to the Teeth* 3rd ed. Copenhagen: Munksgaard Publishers, 1993: 495-516.

2. ANDREASEN JO. Management of soft tissue trauma and alveolar fractures. In: GUTMANN JL, HARRISON JW, eds. *Proceedings of the International Conference on Oral Trauma*. Illinois: American Association of Endodontists Endowment & Memorial Foundation, 1986: 147-54.

3. ZALLEN RD, BLACK SL. Antibiotic therapy in oral and maxillofacial surgery. *J Oral Surg* 1976; 34: 349-51.

4. GOLDBERG MH. Antibiotics and oral and oral-cutaneous lacerations. *J Oral Surg* 1965; 23: 117-22.

5. PATERSON JA, CARDO VA, STRATIGOS GT. An examination of antibiotic prophylaxis in oral and maxillofacial surgery. *J Oral Surg* 1970; 28: 753-9.

6. OSBON DB. Early treatment of soft tissue injuries of the face. *J Oral Surg* 1969; 27: 480-7.

7. LILLY GE. Reaction of oral tissues to suture materials. *Oral Surg Oral Med Oral Pathol* 1968; 26: 128-33.

8. LILLY GE, ARMSTRONG JH, SALEM JE, CUTCHER JL. Reaction of oral tissues to suture materials. Part II. *Oral Surg Oral Med Oral Pathol* 1968; 26: 592-9.

9. LILLY GE, SALEM JE, ARMSTRONG JH, CUTCHER JL. Reaction of oral tissues to suture materials. Part III. *Oral Surg Oral Med Oral Pathol* 1969; 28: 432-8.

10. LILLY GE, CUTCHER JL, JONES JC, ARMSTRONG JH. Reaction of oral tissues to suture materials. Part IV. *Oral Surg Oral Med Oral Pathol* 1972; 33: 152-7.

11. KÁCLOVÁ J, JANOÚSKOVÁ, M. Etude expérimentale sur la réaction des tissus de la cavité buccale aux différents matériaux de suture en chirurgie. *Med Hyg (Geneve)* 1965; 23: 1239.

12. CASTELLI WA, NASJLETI CE, CAFFESSE RE, DIAZ-PEREZ R. Gingival response to silk, cotton, and nylon suture materials. *Oral Surg Oral Med Oral Pathol* 1978; 45: 179-85.

13. WALLACE WR, MAXWELL GR, CAVALARIS CJ. Comparison of polyglycolic acid suture to

black silk, chromic, and plain catgut in human oral tissues. *J Oral Surg* 1970; 28: 739-46.

14. RACEY GL, WALLACE WR, CAVALARIS CJ, MARQUARD JV. Comparison of a polyglycolic-polyactic acid suture to black silk and plain catgut in human oral tissues. *J Oral Surg* 1978; 36: 766-70.

15. BERGENHOLZ A, ISAKSSON B. Tissue reactions in the oral mucosa to catgut, silk, and mersilene sutures. *Odontol Revy* 1967; 18: 237-50.

BIBLIOGRAPHY

Index

A

Abrasion, see Soft tissue wounds
Acid-etch splint, 67, 91, 119, 135
Acid-etch technique, 25
Alveolar process fracture
  diagnosis, 135
  essentials, 140
  follow-up, 140
  pathogenesis, 134
  periodontal healing, 140
  prognosis, 140
  pulp healing, 140
  radiographic diagnosis, 135
  repositioning, 135
  splinting, 135
  treatment, 135
Anachoresis, 119
Ankylosis, 19, 118, 128
  after replantation, 128
  transient, 119
Ankylosis related resorption, 118, 179
Antibiotic therapy, 20, 120, 151, 158
Apical diameter, importance of, 119
Apical foramen, 119
Apical lock, 91, 138
Asphalt tattoos, 162
Avulsion, see also Replantation
  diagnosis, 119
  pathogenesis, 114
  primary dentition, 152
  replantation procedure, 119
  splinting, 120
  treatment, 119

B

Bacteria, role in healing
  complications after avulsion, 117
  crown fracture, 24
  dentin exposure, 24
  luxation injury, 91
  pulp exposure, 35
  replantation, 117
  root fracture, 66
  soft tissue wounds, 157

Battered child syndrome, 12
Bisecting angle exposure, 14
Bonding of crown fragment, 29
Bone resorption, root fracture, 67
Brain concussion, 12

C

Calcium hydroxide
  arrest of root resorption, 122
  root canal dressing, 122
Cleansing procedures
  avulsed teeth, 120
  soft tissue wounds, 157
Clinical examination of the traumatized patient, 12
Clinical examination forms, 173-176
Clinical findings, luxation injuries, 178
Contusion, see Soft tissue wounds
Completed root development and trauma, 82, 83, 99, 100, 111, 129, 130
Complicated crown fracture, see crown fracture
Complicated crown-root fracture, see Crown-root fracture
Composite resin build-up, 28
Composite resin, choice of, 28
Composite technique, 28
Concussion
  diagnosis, 80
  essentials, 84
  follow-up, 81
  pathogenesis, 78
  periodontal healing, 82
  prognosis, 82
  pulp healing, 82
  splinting, 80
  treatment, 80
Connective tissue healing of root fracture, 66
Crown discoloration, primary dentition, 152
Crown fracture
  complicated, 35
  diagnosis, 23

enamel fractures, 25
enamel dentin fractures, 25
  essentials, 44
  follow-up, 42
  infractions, 13
  pathogenesis, 22
  primary dentition, 146
  prognosis, 42
  pulpal healing, 42
  treatment, 25
Crown fragment, reattachment of, 29
Crown-root fracture
  cost-benefit of treatment, 50
  diagnosis, 49
  essentials, 61
  follow-up, 58
  gingivectomy, 52
  orthodontic extrusion, 54
  osteotomy, 52
  pathogenesis, 49
  primary dentition, 146
  prognosis, 58
  radiographic diagnosis, 49
  removal of fragment, 51
  surgical extrusion, 52
  treatment, 50

D

Damage of permanent tooth germ, 143
Deciduous tooth injuries, see primary tooth injuries
Dentin callus, tooth fracture, 65
Dentosafe®, 120
Developmental disturbances, 153
Displacement of tooth germ, 146
Displacement of primary tooth, 143
Disturbances in odontogenesis, 153, 154

E

Electrometric sensibility testing, see Sensibility testing
Emergency records, 173-179

Enamel dentin fracture, treatment, 25
Enamel fractures
  diagnosis, 25
  treatment, 25
Enamel hypoplasia, 143
Enamel opacity, 143
Endodontic treatment
  coronal fragment after root fracture, 72
  crown-root fracture, 54
  extrusive luxation, 98
  intrusive luxation, 107
  lateral luxation, 98
  replantation, 120, 125
  root fracture, 72
Essentials
  alveolar process fracture, 140
  concussion, 84
  crown fracture, 44
  crown-root fractures, 61
  examination of traumatized patient, 16
  extrusive luxation, 101
  intrusive luxation, 112
  lateral luxation, 101
  primary tooth injuries, 155
  replantation, 128
  root fracture, 74
  soft tissue wounds, 171
  subluxation, 84
  treatment principles, 20
  wound healing, 20
Examination
  alveolar process fracture, 135
  avulsion, 119
  concussion, 80
  crown-root fracture, 49
  extrusive luxation, 90
  form, 173
  intrusion, 105
  lateral luxation, 91
  primary tooth injuries, 145
  root fracture, 65
  soft tissue wounds, 156
  subluxation, 80
  traumatized patient, 12
Exarticulation, see Avulsion and Replantation

External inflammatory root resorption, see Inflammatory root resorption
Extraalveolar handling of avulsed tooth, 119
Extraalveolar period, 119, 130
Extraction, primary tooth injuries, 148, 150, 151
Extrusion
orthodontic, see Orthodontic extrusion
surgical, see Surgical extrusion
Extrusive luxation
diagnosis, 90
essentials, 101
follow-up, 98
healing events, 91
pathogenesis, 86
periodontal healing, 98
primary dentition, 147
pulp healing, 98
radiographic diagnosis, 88
repositioning, 90
root resorption, 99
splinting, 90
treatment, 91

F
Fixation, see Splinting
Fixation period, 179
Flexible splint, 20, 92, 96, 121
Fluoride treatment before replantation, 127
Follicle invasion
after intrusive luxation, 143, 145, 148
after lateral luxation, 147
Follow-up procedures
alvealar process fracture, 140
concussion, 81
crown fracture, 38
crown-root fractures, 58
extrusive luxation, 98
intrusive luxation, 111
lateral luxation, 98
primary tooth injuries, 153
replantation, 127
root fracture, 67
subluxation, 81
synopsis, 179
Foreign bodies
clinical diagnosis, 158
radiographic diagnosis, 164
removal of, 158
Fracture of the alveolar process, see Alveolar process fracture
Fracture of the socket wall, 120

G
Gingival reattachment after replantation, 115

Gingival wounds
abrasions, 159
antibiotic treatment, 158
contusion, 160
diagnosis, 159
essentials, 171
foreign bodies, 159
healing events, 158
laceration, 159
pathogenesis, 159
repositioning, 159
suturing, 159
tetanus prophylaxis, 159
treatment, 159
Gingivectomy
crown-root fracture, 52
Glass ionomer cement, 25
Granulation tissue, interposition of in root fracture healing, 66

H
Hard tissue barrier, crown fracture, 37
Hard tissue, root fracture healing, 65
Healing events
extrusive luxation, 91
intrusive luxation, 105
lateral luxation, 91
replantation, 115
root fracture, 65
Hertwig's epithelial root sheath, luxation injury, 91

I
Immature root formation and trauma, 82, 83, 99, 100, 111, 129, 130
Infection, see bacteria and healing complications
Infection related resorption, 98, 117
Inflammatory root resorption, 98, 117
Infractions, diagnosis, 13
Interposition of connective tissue, root fracture healing, 66
Intrusive luxation
diagnosis, 105
essentials, 112
follow-up, 110
healing events, 104
orthodontic extrusion, 107
pathogenesis, 104
percussion test, 105
periodontal healing, 111
primary dentition, 148
prognosis, 110
pulp healing, 111
root resorption, 110
treatment, 107

L
Laceration, see Soft tissue wounds
Lateral luxation
diagnosis, 90

essentials, 101
follow-up, 98
healing events, 91
pathogenesis, 87
periodontal healing, 100
primary dentition, 147
pulp healing, 100
radiographic diagnosis, 89
root resorption, 100
splinting, 94
treatment, 91
Lip wounds
antibiotic treatment, 158
cleansing, 157
debridement, 157
diagnosis, 162
foreign bodies, 158, 164
healing events, 157
pathogenesis, 157, 166
repositioning, 159, 166
suturing, 159, 166
tetanus prophylaxis, 158
treatment, 162
Local anesthetic, 89, 96, 137, 150, 166
Luxation of the permanent tooth germ, 145
Luxation injuries, synopsis of clinical and radiographic findings, 178

M
Malformation of permanent tooth germ, 143
Marginal breakdown, transient, 98
Mature root formation, see Completed root formation
Milk as storage medium, 119
Mixed dentition, anatomy of, 142
Mobility testing, 13

N
Non-healing after root fracture due to infection, 66

O
Observation period after trauma, 179
Occlusal radiographic exposure, 14, 88, 89
Odontogenesis after injury, 143
Oral hygiene after trauma, 98
Orthodontic extrusion
of crown-root fractures, 54
of intruded teeth, 107
Osteotomy
crown-root fracture, 52

P
Partial pulpotomy
clinical procedure, 35
indication, 35

Pathogenesis
alveolar process fracture, 134
avulsion, 114
concussion, 78
crown fracture, 22
crown-root fractures, 48
extrusive luxation, 86
intrusive luxation, 104
lateral luxation, 87
primary tooth injuries, 143
root fracture, 64
soft tissue wounds, 156
subluxation, 79
Penetrating lip lesion, see Soft tissue wounds
Penicillin, 120, 151, 159
Percussion test, 13, 105
Periapical radiolucency, 107, 127
Periodontal healing
alveolar process fracture, 140
concussion, 82
extrusive luxation, 99
general, 18
intrusive luxation, 111
lateral luxation, 100
replantation, 129, 130
subluxation, 83
Photographic registration, 15
Physiologic saline as storage medium, 119
Primary tooth injuries
avulsion, 152
crown fractures, 146
crown-root fractures, 146
diagnosis, 145
essentials, 155
extraction, 148
extrusion, 147
follow-up, 153
intrusion, 148
lateral luxation, 148
pathogenesis, 143
prognosis, 153
pulp necrosis, 153
radiographic examination, 144
replantation, 152
root fractures, 147
treatment, 146
Prognosis of
alveolar process fracture, 140
concussion, 84
crown fracture, 42
crown-root fracture, 58
extrusive luxation, 98
intrusive luxation, 110
lateral luxation, 98
primary tooth injuries, 153
replantation, 129, 130
root fracture, 74
subluxation, 84
Progressive root resorption, see Ankylosis and Inflammatory resorption

INDEX

Prophylactic pulp extirpation, 110, 120
Pulpal revascularization
    after replantation, 116
    after root fracture, 65
    general, 18
Pulp canal obliteration
    root fracture, 66
    sign of previous injury, 13
Pulp capping, 35
Pulp exposure, 35
    and bonding of crown fragment, 39
    healing events, 35
    treatment, 37
Pulp extirpation, see Endodontic treatment
Pulp healing
    alveolar process fracture, 139
    concussion, 82
    crown fracture, 42
    extrusive luxation, 99
    intrusive luxation, 111
    lateral luxation, 100
    partial pulpotomy, 43
    pulp capping, 43
    replantation, 129
    root fracture, 75
    subluxation, 83
Pulp infection after replantation, 124
Pulp necrosis after dental trauma, 42, 43, 75, 82, 83, 99, 100, 111, 129, 130, 139
Pulpotomy
    indication, 35
Pulp survival, see Pulpal healing
Pulp testing, see Sensibility testing

R
Radiographic examination
    alveolar process fracture, 135
    concussion, 80
    crown-root fracture, 49
    extrusive luxation, 88
    general, 14
    lateral luxation, 89
    primary tooth injuries, 144
    root fracture, 65
    subluxation, 80
    traumatic dental injuries, 14
Radiographic findings, luxation injuries, 178
Radiographic guidelines of root fracture healing, 67
Reattachment of crown fragment, 29
Recall schedule, 177
Record for acute dental trauma, 173-177

Re-eruption
    intrusive luxation permanent teeth, 107
    primary dentition, 148
Regional anesthetic, 89, 96, 137, 150, 166
Reimplantation, see Replantation
Removal of coronal fragment, crown-root fracture, 51
Repair related resorption, 116
Replacement root resorption, see Ankylosis
Replantation
    endodontic treatment, 122
    essentials, 131
    fluoride treatment of root surface, 127
    follow-up, 127
    gingival attachment, 115
    healing events, 115
    periodontal healing, 129
    primary dentition, 152
    procedure, 119
    prognosis, 128
    pulp extirpation, 122
    pulp healing, 129
    splinting, 120
Repositioning after
    avulsion, 119
    alveolar process fracture, 135
    extrusive luxation, 91
    lateral luxation, 91
    primary dentition, 146
    root fracture, 67
Root fracture
    diagnosis, 65
    endodontic treatment, 72
    essential, 74
    follow-up, 67
    healing complications, 72
    healing events, 65
    pathogenesis, 64
    primary dentition, 147
    pulp extirpation, 72
    pulp healing, 75
    prognosis, 74
    radiographic diagnosis, 65
    treatment, 67
Root resorption
    after replantation, 116
    extrusive luxation, 99
    inflammatory, 117
    intrusive luxation, 110
    lateral luxation, 100
    replacement, 118
    root fracture, 67
    surface resorption, 116

S
Saliva as storage medium, 119
Sensibility testing
    at time of injury, 14
    concussion, 80
    extrusion, 90, 98
    lateral luxation, 90, 98
    reliability of, 13
    root fracture, 67
    subluxation, 81
Sodium fluoride solution in replantation, 127
Soft diet, 80
Soft tissue wounds
    abrasion, 159, 162
    anatomy, 157
    antibiotic treatment, 158
    cleansing, 157
    contusion, 159
    debridement, 157
    diagnosis, 156
    essentials, 170
    foreign bodies, 158
    healing events, 157
    laceration, 159
    pathogenesis, 156
    repositioning of tissue, 159
    suturing, 159
    tetanus prophylaxis, 158
    treatment, 159, 162, 169
Splinting of
    alveolar process fracture, 135
    concussion, 80
    extrusive luxation, 91
    intrusive luxation, 107
    lateral luxation, 91
    principles, 20
    replantation, 119
    root fracture, 67
    subluxation, 80
Splinting material, 93
Splint removal, 67, 91, 119, 135, 179
Spontaneous re-eruption
    intrusion, permanent dentition, 107
    intrusion, primary dentition, 148
Stage of root development, 82, 83, 99, 100, 111, 129, 130
Storage conditions before replantation, 119
Storage medium before replantation, 119
Storage period
    of teeth before replantation, 119
    periodontal healing after replantation, 130
    pulp healing after replantation, 130
Subluxation
    diagnosis, 80
    essentials, 84

follow-up, 81
pathogenesis, 78
periodontal healing, 83
prognosis, 84
pulp healing, 83
splinting, 80
treatment, 80
Surface root resorption, 116
Surgical extrusion, crown-root fractures, 54

T
Temporization, crown fracture, 29
Tetanus prophylaxis, 120, 158
Tissue culture media, 119
Tooth germ,
    damage to, 143
    displacement, 143, 145
Transient ankylosis, see Ankylosis
Transient marginal breakdown, 98
Treatment
    alveolar process fracture, 135
    avulsion, 119
    concussion, 80
    crown fractures, 25
    crown-root fractures, 50
    extrusive luxation, 91
    intrusive luxation, 107
    lateral luxation, 91
    principles, 19
    primary tooth injuries, 146
    root fracture, 67
    subluxation, 80

U
Uncomplicated crown fracture, see Grown fracture, uncomplicated
Uncomplicated crown-root fracture, see Crown-root fracture

W
Viaspan®, 120
White or yellow-brown discoloration of enamel, 143
White or yellow-brown discoloration of enamel with circular enamel hypoplasia, 143
Wound healing after dental injury, 18

Y
Yellow-brown discoloration of enamel, see White or yellow-brown discoloration og enamel, 143

Z
Zinc oxide-eugenol, 25

188